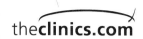

MEDICAL CLINICS
OF NORTH AMERICA

Emergencies in the Outpatient Setting: Part II

GUEST EDITORS
Robert L. Rogers, MD
Joseph P. Martinez, MD

May 2006 • Volume 90 • Number 3

SAUNDERS

An Imprint of Elsevier, Inc.
PHILADELPHIA LONDON TORONTO MONTREAL SYDNEY TOKYO

W.B. SAUNDERS COMPANY
A Division of Elsevier Inc.

1600 John F. Kennedy Boulevard • Suite 1800 • Philadelphia, Pennsylvania 19103-2899

http://www.theclinics.com

MEDICAL CLINICS OF NORTH AMERICA	**Volume 90, Number 3**
May 2006	**ISSN 0025-7125**
Editor: Rachel Glover	**ISBN 1-4160-3673-3**

The ideas and opinions expressed in *Medical Clinics of North America* do not necessarily reflect those of the Publisher. The Publisher does not assume any responsibility for any injury and/or damage to persons or property arising out of or related to any use of the material contained in this periodical. The reader is advised to check the appropriate medical literature and the product information currently provided by the manufacturer of each drug to be administered to verify the dosage, the method and duration of administration, or contraindications. It is the responsibility of the treating physician or other health care professional, relying on independent experience and knowledge of the patient, to determine drug dosages and the best treatment for the patient. Mention of any product in this issue should not be construed as endorsement by the contributors, editors, or the Publisher of the product or manufacturers' claims.

Medical Clinics of North America (ISSN 0025-7125) is published bimonthly by W.B. Saunders, 360 Park Avenue South, New York, NY 10010-1710. Business and editorial offices: 1600 John F. Kennedy Boulevard, Suite 1800, Philadelphia, PA 19103-2899. Accounting and circulation offices: 6277 Sea Harbor Drive, Orlando, FL 32887-4800. Periodicals postage paid at New York, NY, and additional mailing offices. Subscription prices are USD 145 per year for US individuals, USD 260 per year for US institutions, USD 75 per year for US students, USD 185 per year for Canadian individuals, USD 330 per year for Canadian institutions, USD 210 per year for international individuals, USD 330 per year for international institutions and USD 110 per year for Canadian and foreign students/residents. To receive student/resident rate, orders must be accompanied by name of affiliated institution, date of term, and the *signature* of program/residency coordinator on institution letterhead. Orders will be billed at individual rate until proof of status is received. Foreign air speed delivery is included in all *Clinics* subscription prices. All prices are subject to change without notice. POSTMASTER: Send address changes to *Medical Clinics of North America*, Elsevier Periodicals Customer Service, 6277 Sea Harbor Drive, Orlando, FL 32887-4800. **Customer Service: 1-800-654-2452 (US). From outside of the USA, call (+1) 407-345-1000. E-mail: hhspcs@harcourt.com.**

Reprints. For copies of 100 or more, of articles in this publication, please contact the Commercial Reprints Department, Elsevier Inc., 360 Park Avenue South, New York, New York 10010-1710. Tel.: (+1) (212) 633-3813; Fax: (+1) (212) 462-1935; E-mail: reprints@elsevier.com.

Medical Clinics of North America is also published in Spanish by McGraw-Hill Interamericana Editores S. A., P.O. Box 5-237, 06500 Mexico, D.F., Mexico.

Medical Clinics of North America is covered in *Index Medicus, Current Contents, ASCA, Excerpta Medica, Science Citation Index,* and *ISI/BIOMED.*

Printed in the United States of America.

GOAL STATEMENT

The goal of *Medical Clinics of North America* is to keep practicing physicians up to date with current clinical practice by providing timely articles reviewing the state of the art in patient care.

ACCREDITATION

The *Medical Clinics of North America* is planned and implemented in accordance with the Essential Areas and Policies of the Accreditation Council for Continuing Medical Education (ACCME) through the joint sponsorship of the University of Virginia School of Medicine and Elsevier. The University of Virginia School of Medicine is accredited by the ACCME to provide continuing medical education for physicians.

The University of Virginia School of Medicine designates this educational activity for a maximum of 90 category 1 credits per year, 15 category 1 credits per issue, toward the AMA Physician's Recognition Award. Each physician should claim only those credits that he/she actually spent in the activity.

The American Medical Association has determined that physicians not licensed in the US who participate in this CME activity are eligible for AMA PRA category 1 credit.

Category 1 credit can be earned by reading the text material, taking the CME examination online at *http://www.theclinics.com/home/cme*, and completing the evaluation. After taking the test, you will be required to review any and all incorrect answers. Following completion of the test and evaluation, your credit will be awarded and you may print your certificate.

FACULTY DISCLOSURE/CONFLICT OF INTEREST

The University of Virginia School of Medicine, as an ACCME accredited provider, endorses and strives to comply with the Accreditation Council for Continuing Medical Education (ACCME) Standards of Commercial Support, Commonwealth of Virginia statutes, University of Virginia policies and procedures, and associated federal and private regulations and guidelines on the need for disclosure and monitoring of proprietary and financial interests that may affect the scientific integrity and balance of content delivered in continuing medical education activities under our auspices.

The University of Virginia School of Medicine requires that all CME activities accredited through this institution be developed independently and be scientifically rigorous, balanced and objective in the presentation/discussion of its content, theories and practices.

All authors/editors participating in an accredited CME activity are expected to disclose to the readers relevant financial relationships with commercial entities occurring within the past 12 months (such as grants or research support, employee, consultant, stock holder, member of speakers bureau, etc.). The University of Virginia School of Medicine will employ appropriate mechanisms to resolve potential conflicts of interest to maintain the standards of fair and balanced education to the reader. Questions about specific strategies can be directed to the Office of Continuing Medical Education, University of Virginia School of Medicine, Charlottesville, Virginia.

The authors/editors listed below have identified no professional or financial affiliations for themselves or their spouse/partner:
John S. Flanigan, MD; Rachel Glover, Acquistions Editor; Luis H. Haro, MD; Erik P. Hess, MD; Mark D. Kelemen, MD, MSc, FACC; Paul Kleutz, MD; Joseph P. Martinez, MD; Robert L. Rogers, MD, FAAEM, FACEP, FACP; Jose Santana, MD; Joseph R. Shiber, MD; David Vitberg, MD; Michael E. Winters, MD; and, Jeffrey Zilberstein, MD.

The authors/editors listed below identified the following professional or financial affiliations for themselves or their spouse/partner:
Wyatt W. Decker, MD is on the speakers' bureau for Given Imaging, LLC, INrange Pharmaceuticals, and Boston Scientific.
Mark H. Flasar, MD has an educational grant from Centocor.
Eric Goldberg, MD is on the speakers' bureau for Given Imaging, LLC, INrange Pharmaceuticals, and Boston Scientific.

Disclosure of Discussion of non-FDA approved uses for pharmaceutical products and/or medical devices:
The University of Virginia School of Medicine, as an ACCME provider, requires that all faculty presenters identify and disclose any "off label" uses for pharmaceutical and medical device products. The University of Virginia School of Medicine recommends that each physician fully review all the available data on new products or procedures prior to instituting them with patients.

TO ENROLL

To enroll in the Medical Clinics of North America Continuing Medical Education program, call customer service at 1-800-654-2452 or visit us online at *http://www.theclinics.com/home/cme*. The CME program is available to subscribers for an additional fee of USD 205.

FORTHCOMING ISSUES

RECENT ISSUES

GUEST EDITORS

ROBERT L. ROGERS, MD, FAAEM, FACEP, FACP, Assistant Professor (Surgery), Division of Emergency Medicine; Director, Undergraduate Medical Education; and Associate Residency Director, Emergency Medicine, University of Maryland School of Medicine, Baltimore, Maryland

JOSEPH P. MARTINEZ, MD, Assistant Professor (Surgery), Division of Emergency Medicine, University of Maryland School of Medicine; and Assistant Medical Director, Adult Emergency Department, University of Maryland Medical System, Baltimore, Maryland

CONTRIBUTORS

WYATT W. DECKER, MD, Chair, Department of Emergency Medicine, Mayo Clinic; and Associate Professor (Emergency Medicine), Mayo Clinic College of Medicine, Rochester, Minnesota

JOHN S. FLANIGAN, MD, Assistant Professor (Surgery), Division of Emergency Medicine, University of Maryland School of Medicine, Baltimore, Maryland

MARK H. FLASAR, MD, Clinical Instructor (Medicine), Division of Gastroenterology and Hepatology, Department of Medicine, University of Maryland Medical Center, Baltimore, Maryland

ERIC GOLDBERG, MD, Assistant Professor, Division of Gastroenterology and Hepatology, Department of Medicine, University of Maryland Medical Center, Baltimore, Maryland

LUIS H. HARO, MD, Consultant, Department of Emergency Medicine, Mayo Clinic; and Instructor (Emergency Medicine), Mayo Clinic College of Medicine, Rochester, Minnesota

ERIK P. HESS, MD, Critical Care Medicine Fellow, Division of Critical Care, Department of Medicine, Mayo Clinic, Rochester, Minnesota

MARK D. KELEMEN, MD, MSc, FACC, Associate Professor (Medicine), Division of Cardiology, University of Maryland School of Medicine, Baltimore, Maryland

PAUL KLUETZ, MD, Resident, Department of Medicine, University of Maryland Medical Center, Baltimore, Maryland

JOSE SANTANA, MD, Senior Resident, Department of Emergency Medicine, East Carolina University, Greenville, North Carolina

JOSEPH R. SHIBER, MD, Clinical Assistant Professor, Departments of Medicine and Emergency Medicine; and Director, Emergency Medicine–Internal Medicine Combined Residency, East Carolina University, Greenville, North Carolina

DAVID VITBERG, MD, Chief Resident, Combined Program of Internal Medicine and Emergency Medicine, University of Maryland School of Medicine, Baltimore, Maryland

MICHAEL E. WINTERS, MD, Instructor, Department of Medicine and Division of Emergency Medicine, Department of Surgery, University of Maryland School of Medicine; and Associate Program Director, Combined Internal Medicine and Emergency Medicine Residency Program, University of Maryland Medical Center, Baltimore, Maryland

JEFFREY ZILBERSTEIN, MD, Resident, Combined Internal Medicine and Emergency Medicine Residency Program, University of Maryland Medical Center, Baltimore, Maryland

CONTENTS

ELSEVIER
SAUNDERS

THE MEDICAL
CLINICS
OF NORTH AMERICA

Med Clin N Am 90 (2006) xi–xii

Preface

Emergencies in the Outpatient Setting: Part II

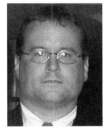
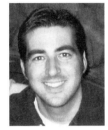

Robert L. Rogers, MD   Joseph P. Martinez, MD
Guest Editors

The evaluation of patients in the outpatient setting frequently results in the need to transport them to the emergency department (ED) for definitive diagnosis and management. Many chief complaints and specific disease entities are more easily managed in the ED due to the availability of airway and resuscitation equipment and access to specialty consultant care. Any discussion of emergent patient presentations would be remiss without discussing the obvious fact that many of the urgent and emergent conditions that develop in our patients are difficult to take care of in the office.

Primary care providers who see patients in the outpatient arena should be fully prepared to treat and stabilize ill patients to a higher level of care prior to transport. Furthermore, these providers must have concrete knowledge as to what conditions should be managed in the ED and what complaints and entities are best handled in the office to avoid unnecessary transport and ED overcrowding. Finally, there is a need for the primary care physician to be familiar with and understand subtle and atypical presentations of disease as well as the classic appearance. Although many patients will be quickly transported to the ED for stabilization, diagnosis, and admission, it is the outpatient physician's obligation to recognize whether a potential life threat exists in the first place.

The main goal of Part II of this double issue is to review some common urgent and emergent conditions that present to primary care offices. Topics of discussion include, (1) what conditions can and should be treated in the office without necessitating patient transport; (2) what entities require urgent or emergent transfer to the ED; (3) how to prepare your office for an emergency;

and (4) what some of the "can't miss" entities could be that primary care physicians should be familiar with. With these in mind, Part II focuses on topics that are common and potentially life- or limb-threatening. Our goal is to provide a useful resource for the outpatient physician on what to do when faced with certain urgent and emergent patient complaints and presentations.

In the pages that follow, several common patient complaints and presentations will be discussed as they relate to how they are handled differently in the outpatient versus inpatient setting. The authors acknowledge that several of the articles included in this double issue cover topics that, on the surface, appear to be only appropriate for ED evaluation. For example, why were we compelled to discuss arrhythmias, pulmonary embolism, myocardial infarction, aortic dissection, spinal cord compression, or extremity fractures? Are any of these entities taken care of in the office setting? The answer is a resounding, "No." However, patients with these and numerous other conditions present initially to a primary care provider's office. Outpatient practitioners should be well aware that they are, to some degree, on the front line of patient care as much as emergency physicians, and are poised to make a tremendous difference in the lives of patients who seek medical attention for urgent and emergent problems. Prompt recognition of emergent medical and surgical conditions often starts with simply considering what potential diagnoses may be present and in what setting would be most appropriate for patient care. So, although many of these entities are dismissed from the office as quickly as they entered, it is important to note that the primary care physician can make a difference by being knowledgeable of the acute care issues at hand and working under the assumption that a limb- or life-threat is present until proven otherwise. We hope that Part II of this double issue proves useful in refreshing or providing that very knowledge.

Robert L. Rogers, MD
Assistant Professor (Surgery), Division of Emergency Medicine
Director, Undergraduate Medical Education
Associate Residency Director, Emergency Medicine
University of Maryland School of Medicine
Baltimore, MD, USA

E-mail address: rrogers@medicine.umaryland.edu

Joseph P. Martinez, MD
Assistant Professor (Surgery), Division of Emergency Medicine
University of Maryland School of Medicine

Assistant Medical Director, Adult Emergency Department
University of Maryland Medical System
Baltimore, MD, USA

E-mail address: jmartine@umaryland.edu

ELSEVIER
SAUNDERS

THE MEDICAL
CLINICS
OF NORTH AMERICA

Med Clin N Am 90 (2006) 391–416

Angina Pectoris: Evaluation in the Office

Mark D. Kelemen, MD, MSc*

Division of Cardiology, University of Maryland School of Medicine, Baltimore, MD, USA

Chest pain is one of the most common complaints of patients who are seen in an ambulatory practice. The major early objective in the diagnosis of such patients is to separate noncardiac from cardiac pain. This article reviews the pathogenesis of coronary artery disease (CAD) and its most common clinical symptom, angina pectoris. Coronary heart disease (CHD) caused by atherosclerosis is one of the most common ailments in the Western world and remains the leading nontraumatic cause of disability and death in the United States. An increase in public awareness and health education has lowered CHD mortality by more than 20% in the last 25 years. However, it remains the leading cause of death among both men and women. Patients who have chest pain often seek medical attention. It is essential that physicians know how to respond to such patients to make appropriate diagnostic and therapeutic decisions. In the approach to the patient who has chest pain, a detailed history and physical examination must not be replaced by sophisticated procedures but should allow the physician to select the most appropriate diagnostic tests.

Pathogenesis

The endothelium plays an integral role in the defense against atherosclerosis and in modulating vascular tone and preventing thrombosis in blood vessels. These endothelial functions are affected by the presence of CAD risk factors, even before atherosclerosis is evident. In the earliest stages, circulating monocytes adhere to the endothelial cells (through adhesion molecules) and migrate into the intima of the blood vessel, where they ingest oxidatively modified low-density lipoprotein (LDL) and are trapped as

---
* Division of Cardiology, University of Maryland School of Medicine, 419 West Redwood Street, Suite 550, Baltimore, MD 21201-1734.
  E-mail address: mkelemen@medicine.umaryland.edu

0025-7125/06/$ - see front matter
doi:10.1016/j.mcna.2005.12.002
medical.theclinics.com

foam cells. Collections of foam cells, known as fatty streaks, have been found in early childhood. Foam cells die, leading to the development of a lipid core, and smooth muscle cells are signaled to migrate from the media, destroying the internal elastic lamina of the vessel in the process. Calcification of the plaque occurs early and can be visualized with techniques such as CT and MRI. The arterial wall begins to thicken and remodel. Based on intravascular ultrasonographic studies, the encroachment of plaque into the lumen of a coronary artery is a late process and reflects advanced disease (the arterial cross-sectional area is reduced by 40% before a lesion is visible as luminal narrowing at catheterization).

The progression of atherosclerosis is accelerated by three processes: endothelial dysfunction, inflammation, and thrombosis. The advanced atherosclerotic lesion has a core of lipid and necrotic tissue surrounded by a fibrous cap. This cap contains collagen, and its characteristics are related to the risk of plaque rupture, the most common cause of acute coronary syndromes. Specifically, the thinner the cap, the more likely it is to rupture. Shear stress at the edge or "shoulder" region of a plaque, inflammation at the endothelial surface of the cap, or internal degradation of the cap by enzymes known as metalloproteinases are other major determinants of the likelihood of plaque rupture. A ruptured plaque leads very quickly to thrombus formation. The complete occlusion of a coronary vessel by ruptured plaque manifests as an acute transmural or ST elevation myocardial infarction (ie, STEMI). Nonocclusive thrombus can cause unstable angina or non–ST elevation MI (ie, NSTEMI). Nonocclusive thrombus may not cause symptoms but, instead, may change plaque geometry, leading to rapid plaque growth. Studies have shown that an acute MI may be more likely to occur in an area that was previously not severely narrowed (ie, less than 50% luminal reduction by angiography) than in an area that was more severely narrowed (ie, more than 70% luminal reduction). Narrowing of a coronary artery by 70% or greater is more likely to cause exertional angina. The discordance between plaque severity and the development of acute MI indicates that MI is not simply a mechanical problem.

Most patients who have classic angina by history have fixed atherosclerotic lesions of 70% or more in at least one major coronary artery [1]. However, a 70% stenosis viewed by two-dimensional angiography is associated with a reduction of approximately 90% in cross-sectional area. Angina is cause by a mismatch between myocardial oxygen supply and demand. Oxygen supply is determined by coronary perfusion pressure and coronary vascular resistance. Flow is autoregulated over a wide range of perfusion pressures, and therefore, most of the changes in flow are caused by changes in resistance (ie, vasodilation). However, the coronary bed, beyond a significant flow-limiting stenosis, is typically dilated maximally, so that small increases in demand (eg, increased heart rate and blood pressure during exercise) may result in myocardial ischemia. Demand is related to heart rate, systolic blood pressure, and wall tension. Wall tension is determined by ventricular pressure, cavity size, and wall thickness. Exercise and emotional stress have potent effects on these variables and, not coincidentally, are the common triggers for ischemic chest pain.

Risk factors

Genetic and environmental risk factors influence the development of atherosclerotic heart disease. Research has been targeted at defining the role of these factors in the premature development of CAD. The recognition of risk factors is important especially because they may be modified to prevent disease. Landmark epidemiologic surveys like the Framingham Heart Study helped to define levels of risk for the individual risk factors. Treatment guidelines have been revised recently to include the important interactions between individual risk factors and age. Risk calculators (CHD event risk over 10 years) are available elsewhere [2,3].

The 27th Bethesda Conference [4] was designed to bring attention to specific patients who are at high-risk for the development of CAD events. The findings have been incorporated into the National Cholesterol Education Program (NCEP) Detection, Evaluation and Treatment of High Blood Cholesterol in Adults (adult treatment panel [ATP]-III) [5]. The concepts of "risk" and "risk factor" are important in understanding and using the guidelines. The Bethesda Conference outlines four categories of risk based on observational studies and efficacy studies (clinical trials) (Box 1).

Category 1 risk factors for which interventions have been proven to reduce the risk of CHD events, include smoking, LDL cholesterol, high saturated fat diet, hypertension, LVH, and "thrombogenic factor," which are unnamed but reflect a reduction of risk with the use of aspirin. Category 2 risk factors, for which interventions are likely to lower CHD risk, include diabetes mellitus, physical inactivity, HDL cholesterol, elevated triglycerides, small, dense LDL particles, obesity, and postmenopausal status in women. Since the publication of these findings, diabetes has been reclassified as a CHD "risk equivalent" based on data suggesting that diabetic patients who do not have known CAD have similar survival to nondiabetic patients who have suffered a myocardial infarction. The ATP-III guidelines [5] focus attention on the "metabolic syndrome" that incorporates abdominal obesity, atherogenic dyslipidemia (elevated triglycerides, small LDL particles, low HDL cholesterol), elevated blood pressure, insulin resistance (with or without glucose intolerance), and prothrombotic and proinflammatory states. Patients who have this syndrome are now appropriately targeted for intensive lipid modification. HDL cholesterol, with the publication of the Veterans Affairs High-density Lipoprotein Intervention Trial (ie, VA-HIT) [6], may now rightly be considered a category 1 risk factor because the intervention to raise HDL cholesterol level with gemfibrozil reduced the incidence of cardiovascular events. Although postmenopausal status

---

Box 1. Cardiovascular risk factors

Category 1: risk factors for which interventions have been proven to lower (cardiovascular disease) CVD risk
Cigarette smoking
LDL cholesterol
High fat/cholesterol diet
Hypertension
Left ventricular hypertrophy (LVH)
Thrombogenic factors (as affected by aspirin)

Category 2: risk factors for which interventions are likely to lower CVD risk
Diabetes mellitus
Physical Inactivity
High-density lipoprotein (HDL) cholesterol[a]
Triglycerides
Small, dense LDL particle size
Obesity
Postmenopausal status (women)

Category 3: risk factors associated with increased CVD risk that, if modified, might lower risk
Psychosocial factors
Lipoprotein(a)
Homocysteine
Oxidative stress
No alcohol consumption

Category 4: risk factors associated with increased risk but which cannot be modified
Age
Male sex
Low socioeconomic status
Family history of early onset CVD

---

[a] May now be considered a category-1 risk factor; see text.
Adapted from Fuster V, Pearson TA, Co-Chairs. 27th Bethesda conference: matching the intensity of risk factor management with the hazard for coronary disease events. J Am Coll Cardiol 1996;27(5):957–1047.

---

correctly identifies the risk factor, hormone replacement therapy is now contraindicated for the treatment of women who have CAD or are at high risk for CAD for the purpose of reducing cardiovascular risk. Category 3 risk factors are those that are associated with an increased CAD risk that may, if modified, lower risk. These factors include the so-called putative or emerging risk factors such as depression, lipoprotein a, homocysteine, oxidative stress, and alcohol. Since 1997, this list should be expanded to include inflammatory markers (white blood cell count, high-sensitivity C-reactive protein [CRP] level, soluble adhesion molecules, and chlamydial infection), thrombotic risk factors (plasminogen activator inhibitor-1), and sleep apnea. Coronary calcification measured by electron beam CT [7] can be considered correctly a category 3 risk factor for now but may need to be reclassified (like diabetes) as a CAD risk equivalent because it functionally measures subclinical coronary artery plaque burden. Moderate alcohol consumption may reduce CAD risk. Category 4 risk factors, which are associated with increased risk but cannot be modified, include age, male sex, low socioeconomic status, and a family history of early onset CAD. A positive family history has been defined as a CAD risk factor in a male first-degree relative younger than 55 years of age or in a female first-degree relative younger than 65 years of age. These factors are usually taken into consideration with the available risk scoring systems.

Diagnosis and history

A careful history is of paramount importance in the diagnosis of angina and can be as effective as exercise testing in predicting the extent of underlying coronary artery disease [8]. The discomfort of myocardial ischemia may be described variously by patients; many do not describe it as a pain, so it is often more effective to ask the patient to describe the discomfort. Some patients describe it as a squeezing, crushing, burning, or smothering sensation, whereas others describe a shortness of breath or simply a feeling of heaviness. Some patients may use a Levine's sign, a clenched fist in the middle of the chest, to describe the discomfort. Rarely is the patient able to point with one finger to the location; so when pain can be localized in this way, it is likely to be noncardiac in origin. A sharp pain is unlikely to have a cardiac origin, but the patient should be asked to characterize it further. In some regions of the United States, "sharp" means severe rather than knifelike or piercing.

Angina, as described classically, begins and ends gradually, usually over 2 to 5 minutes, and is steady in character, although it can occasionally wax and wane. The anginal threshold may be lower in the morning. If ischemic pain continues for over 20 minutes, myocardial infarction is likely. The discomfort is midline and substernal; it often radiates to the shoulder, arm, hand or fingers, usually to the left. Radiation down the inside of the arm into the fingers supplied by the ulnar nerve is a classic sign. Pain also may radiate into the neck, the lower (but not the upper) jaw, or the intrascapular region. Occasionally, the patient may have pain only in a referred location and experience no chest discomfort at all. An "anginal equivalent" refers to a discomfort limited to the site typically noted in secondary radiation of pain. Dyspnea may be an anginal equivalent in older individuals but should be centrally located; the dyspnea of a pulmonary cause is not localized. Uncomfortable arm heaviness may represent angina. Gaseous distension, belching, nausea, and indigestion are common accompanying symptoms. Chest pain accompanied by severe diaphoresis is worrisome but is not always caused by cardiac ischemia.

The Canadian Cardiovascular Society (CCS) classification system [9] predicts the extent of CAD and risk of ischemic events. CCS class I angina occurs with strenuous, rapid, or prolonged exertion but not with ordinary physical activity. Class II is defined as a slight limitation of ordinary activity. Angina occurs on walking or climbing stairs rapidly, walking uphill, walking or stair climbing after meals, in cold or wind exposure, or under emotional stress. Class III angina has marked limitations of ordinary physical activity. Angina occurs on walking one or two blocks on a level surface and climbing one flight of stairs in normal conditions and at a normal pace. Class IV, the most severe, is the inability to carry on any physical activity without discomfort, and anginal symptoms may be present at rest.

A major feature of the history is the identification of precipitating and aggravating factors. The single most important diagnostic feature of the discomfort of myocardial ischemia is a predictable relationship to exertion, emotional stress, or other situations that increase myocardial oxygen demand or reduce supply. The cause of atypical pain, pain in an unusual location or of an unusual character, may be clarified by this relationship. Pain that is experienced at rest, if it is caused by ischemia, suggests unstable angina or myocardial infarction. Anxiety and mental stress are important and often overlooked provoking factors in many patients. Myocardial oxygen demand may be increased by anxiety to an extent and duration greater that that produced by exercise, resulting in prolonged pain. Angina is more likely to occur during cold or windy weather because of increased peripheral vascular resistance and consequently increased myocardial work. Sexual intercourse may represent the highest daily energy expenditure in sedentary elderly patients who have subclinical CAD. Sometimes, ischemic discomfort follows a heavy meal, perhaps caused by the shunting of blood to abdominal viscera and because of increased sympathetic tone. Nocturnal angina may be a consequence or manifestation of left ventricular failure or may represent unstable angina. Similarly, patients who describe breathlessness and chest pain with exertion may have angina as a consequence of transient left ventricular failure.

Because angina is caused by a discrepancy between oxygen supply and demand, the relief of pain is achieved by increasing coronary blood flow or decreasing oxygen demand, and angina begins to disappear within minutes thereafter. So-called walk-through angina is uncommon. Most people must stop or at least slow the activity responsible for precipitating the pain before it is relieved. However, it is common for people to resume their activities and walk farther the second time without symptoms; this is known as "preconditioning." A history of relief of pain by sublingual nitroglycerin is also useful. However, the patient must be told that the use of nitroglycerin in this way is a diagnostic trial and that the prescription of nitroglycerin does not necessarily mean coronary artery disease. The relief of chest pain by nitroglycerin is not specific for myocardial ischemia; the pain of esophageal spasm is commonly relieved by nitroglycerin. A placebo effect may relieve chest discomfort from other causes as well.

Physical examination

Physical examination findings in patients who have angina are nonspecific. Particular attention is paid to uncovering circumstantial evidence that would support the diagnosis of coronary artery disease: high blood pressure, evidence of abnormal lipid metabolism such as tendon xanthomas or xanthelesma, fundoscopic changes reflecting long-standing hypertension or diabetes mellitus, or evidence of peripheral vascular disease. A complete cardiovascular examination should include measurement of bilateral blood pressures and auscultation of the carotid, abdominal aorta, and femoral arteries. Aortic stenosis should be excluded, with systolic murmurs (present in 70% of the elderly) confirmed by diminished and delayed pulses (pulsus parvus et tardus) in the carotids or left brachial artery. A focus on auscultation and the character and timing of murmurs will lead to an appropriate referral for echocardiography. If a patient has chest pain in the office, the blood pressure should be taken immediately because hypertension (ischemia) or hypotension (acute heart failure) can be important signs. Furthermore, the presence of a new mitral regurgitation murmur during chest pain may signal extensive ischemia.

Laboratory evaluation, including cardiac biomarkers

The laboratory evaluation of patients presenting with new angina pectoris focuses on evaluating risk factors. Hypertensive patients should have an evaluation of renal function. Diabetic patients should have an assessment of the level of control of blood glucose (ie, hemoglobin A_{1c}). Patients who have impaired glucose tolerance (fasting plasma glucose 100–126) or are suspected of having the metabolic syndrome (abdominal obesity, high triglycerides, hypertension, and low HDL cholesterol) should undergo an oral glucose tolerance test to screen for overt diabetes. The NCEP [5] recommends screening fasting lipid levels in all adults with a measurement of HDL cholesterol. Many practitioners are using advanced lipid testing (ie, LDL particle number and density), but there is no consensus on its use. Similarly, elevated levels of high-sensitivity CRP [10] and B-type natriuretic peptide [11] are associated with prognosis in patients who have angina pectoris but have not yet been incorporated into the guidelines. The measurement of cardiac troponin should be reserved for patients who have suspected acute coronary syndromes.

Electrocardiogram

A 12-lead ECG should be obtained as soon as possible in a patient suspected of having CAD or angina, but in many cases, results may be completely normal. The most reliable ECG sign of chronic ischemic heart disease is a pathologic Q wave, representing previous infarction. Nonspecific ST-T wave changes, abnormalities of conduction (except for LBBB), and arrhythmias do not help establish the diagnosis of myocardial ischemia. ST segment depression with a flat or downward sloping ST segment, however, is indicative of subendocardial ischemia. It is seldom present in the resting ECG of patients who have ischemic heart disease, unless they are experiencing angina at the time the tracing is being recorded. On the other hand, these transient ischemic changes are seen commonly when a patient who has ischemic heart disease is exercised to a point at which chest pain develops. Such ECG changes, appearing with exercise or pain and resolving with rest or with the resolution of pain, strongly indicate myocardial ischemia. Therefore, the necessity of repeating the ECG at rest or after the chest pain has resolved cannot be overemphasized. ST segment elevation during chest pain suggests myocardial infarction or variant angina.

T wave inversion in an ECG taken at rest is a nonspecific finding but can occur after infarction or as a specific transient finding in a patient who has angina. Thus, ECG changes noted during episodes of chest pain not only confirm the diagnosis of myocardial ischemia but also may indicate the extent and location of the ischemic myocardium. As a general rule, the more widespread the changes, the more myocardium is involved.

The differential diagnosis of Q waves on an ECG include previous myocardial infarction, healed myocarditis, an infiltrative myocardial disorder like amyloidosis or sarcoidosis, and pre-excitation (delta wave) from Wolff-Parkinson-White syndrome. Similarly, ST segment elevation in the absence of chest pain is common in the resting ECG of healthy young adults and is caused by rapid or "early" repolarization of the ventricle. This pattern is noted usually in the mid-left chest leads (V_2–V_4) but has also been seen widely. ST segment elevation from pericarditis is diffuse, can be associated with PR segment depression, and has the other usual clinical features. The presence of ST-T abnormalities in an otherwise healthy person is a nonspecific finding and should not be considered confirmation of CAD. There is a high association of left bundle branch block (LBBB) with organic heart disease, especially CAD. Right bundle branch block (RBBB), on the other hand, is present in 0.3% of normal people and is usually a benign, congenital condition. RBBB is rarely a manifestation of CAD.

Differential diagnosis

A complete differential diagnosis of chest pain is outside the scope of this article but can be classified generally as cardiovascular causes and noncardiac causes. The cardiovascular causes include stable and unstable angina, myocardial infarction, pericarditis, aortic dissection (or enlarging aneurysm), pulmonary embolism, and pulmonary hypertension. Noncardiac causes include musculoskeletal disorders, esophageal and other gastrointestinal pain, neuropathic pain including herpes zoster, and anxiety.

Stress testing

The American College of Cardiology (ACC)/American Heart Association (AHA) exercise testing guidelines were updated in 1997 [12]. Patients who have a high likelihood of having CAD by history should be referred directly for cardiac catheterization. Those with a low likelihood of CAD should not undergo exercise testing. Table 1 shows the ACC/AHA criteria for determining the probability of underlying CAD by age, sex, and symptoms. Typical features of angina include the location and character of discomfort, timing of discomfort, and inciting and relieving factors. The ACC/AHA class I recommendation for exercise testing in the diagnosis of CAD is for adult patients who have an intermediate pretest probability of CAD (15%–85%). For patients who are known to have CAD, the guidelines recommend stress testing for those who experience a significant change in clinical status. Absolute and relative contraindications to stress testing are

Table 1
Pretest likelihood of coronary artery disease in symptomatic patients according to age and sex

| | | | Angina | | | |
| | Nonanginal chest pain likelihood (%) | | Atypical likelihood (%) | | Typical likelihood (%) | |
Age (y)	Men	Women	Men	Women	Men	Women
30–39	4	2	34	12	76	26
40–49	13	3	51	22	87	55
50–59	20	7	65	31	93	73
60–69	27	14	72	51	94	86

No data exists for patients <30 y or >69 y, but it can be assumed that prevalence of coronary artery disease increases with age. In a few cases, patients with ages at the extremes of the decades listed may have probabilities slightly outside the high or low range. High indicates 90%; intermediate 10%–90%; low, <10%; and very low, <5%.

Data from Gibbons RJ, Abrams J, Chatterjee K, et al. ACC/AHA 2002 guideline update for the management of patients with chronic stable angina: a report of the American College of Cardiology/American Heart Association Task Force on Practice Guidelines (Committee to update the 1999 guidelines for the management of patients with chronic stable angina). © 2002 American College of Cardiology and American Heart Association. Available at http://www.acc.org/clinical/guidelines/stable/stable.pdf. Accessed January 13, 2006.

outlined in Box 2 [12]. Unstable angina, decompensated heart failure, aortic stenosis, and uncontrolled hypertension are the most common reasons for canceling a test.

The simplest and least expensive test is the exercise treadmill test [13]. Many European countries prefer bicycle stress testing; the routine use of bicycles in the United States is rare. Various protocols have been devised for graded, symptom-limited exercise testing, but all protocols have the same rationale. As cardiac work is increased, myocardial oxygen consumption increases and coronary blood flow must increase. If a fixed coronary obstruction limits changes in blood flow, the patient may experience chest discomfort, and ECG changes (ST segment depression) can occur. Fig. 1 represents a simple algorithm for deciding what type of stress test to recommend. Baseline ECG abnormalities that preclude a simple exercise ECG include pre-excitation (Wolff-Parkinson-White syndrome), electronically paced ventricular rhythm, a resting ST depression greater than 1 mm, and complete left bundle branch block. These patients should be referred for imaging stress tests and their ability to exercise determined. The inability to perform 4 METs or metabolic equivalents of exercise is an independent, poor prognostic sign for long-term outcome. The Duke activity score [12] is useful for predicting exercise ability. The simple question "Can you walk up a flight of stairs carrying laundry or groceries without stopping?"

Box 2. Absolute contraindications to exercise testing

Acute myocardial infarction (<2 d)
High-risk unstable angina
Decompensated heart failure
Uncontrolled cardiac arrhythmias with symptoms or
    hemodynamic compromise
Advanced atrioventricular block
Acute myocarditis or pericarditis
Severe symptomatic aortic stenosis
Severe hypertrophic obstructive cardiomyopathy
Uncontrolled hypertension
Acute systemic illness (pulmonary embolism, aortic dissection)

Relative contraindications can be superseded if the benefits of exercise outweigh the risks. The appropriate timing of testing depends on the level of risk of unstable angina. In the absence of definitive evidence, the committee suggests systolic blood pressure greater than 200 mm Hg and/or diastolic blood pressure greater than 110 mm Hg.

Data from Gibbons RJ, Balady GJ, Beasley FW, et al. ACC/AHA guidelines for exercise testing: a report of the ACC/AHA task force on practice guidelines. J Am Coll Cardiol 1997;30:260–315.

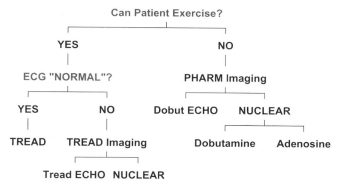

Fig. 1. Algorithm for determining the appropriate stress test (see section "Stress testing"). Dobut, dobutamine; ECHO, echocardiography.

is an excellent discriminator for exercise ability. If the answer is "Yes," treadmill exercise is recommended; if the answer is "No," a pharmacologic stress test with cardiac imaging is recommended. Cost-effectiveness analysis has shown that the choice between nuclear perfusion imaging and echocardiography imaging is so close that the most important factor is the relative expertise of the local laboratories [14].

Radioisotope imaging

Radioisotope imaging can enhance the specificity of stress testing by evaluating myocardial function or flow [15]. Radioisotope imaging can be used in conjunction with either treadmill exercise testing or pharmacologic stress testing, using either dobutamine to increase cardiac work or adenosine or dipyridamole to alter coronary blood flow. Commonly used imaging modalities include radioisotope imaging with thallium-201 (^{201}Tl) or technetium-99m (^{99m}Tc)–based agents (eg, ^{99m}Tc sestamibi). The usefulness of ^{201}Tl as a perfusion tracer is based on its ability to function as an analog of ionic potassium. It is most efficiently extracted by healthy myocardial cells, and uptake is proportional to regional perfusion and myocardial viability. ^{99m}Tc sestamibi has a shorter half-life (6 hours) than ^{201}Tl (73 hours), which allows a larger tracer dose to be administered. This and its higher emission energy make ^{99m}Tc an excellent agent for cardiac imaging. ^{99m}Tc sestamibi is particularly useful in obese patients and in patients who have large breasts (because of the possible attenuation of the radioisotopic images in the area of the anterior myocardium).

Both ^{201}Tl and ^{99m}Tc sestamibi can be used to assess regional myocardial blood flow, either by planar imaging or by single-photon emission CT (SPECT). Imaging usually occurs at two separate times: the stress scan is obtained very shortly after the patient has exercised or received a pharmacologic agent, and the rest scan is obtained either before or several hours after stress. The radioisotope is injected intravenously (IV) at the time of peak exercise (or at the time of peak infusion during a pharmacologic stress test), and scintigraphic images are obtained shortly thereafter, depicting regional myocardial perfusion at the time of peak stress. The rest scan is typically obtained later and shows redistribution of the isotope. Ischemia is indicated by the filling in of a cold spot defined on the stress images (ie, normalization or "redistribution" of a radioisotopic defect), and infarction is indicated by a persisting cold spot or one with only partial redistribution. Fig. 2A demonstrates the standard nomenclature for radioisotope imaging, and Fig. 2B shows the typical coronary artery territories [16].

Radioisotope imaging with stress-gated blood pool scans (multiple gated acquisition [MUGA]) can also be used to assess myocardial ischemia. To allow for continuous imaging during exercise, stress MUGA is performed with the patient exercising on a semirecumbent bicycle. The rationale for this test is the fact that myocardium that becomes ischemic during graded exercise develops regional wall motion abnormalities that can be detected by sequential image analysis. This type of imaging labels the blood pool with a radioisotope and gates image acquisition to the ECG. Right and left ventricular volumes, regional left ventricular wall motion, and global and regional ejection fractions can be measured, both at rest and with stress.

Stress echocardiography

Two-dimensional echocardiography can be used instead of radioisotope scanning to detect areas of regional myocardial dysfunction (as evidenced by a wall motion abnormality) with exercise or pharmacologic stress. Typically, baseline images are first obtained at rest to determine the adequacy of the echocardiographic images. If these images are technically inadequate (ie, because of obesity or obstructive lung disease), then IV contrast agents can be used or the patient should be referred for radioisotope imaging (most laboratories report a 5% failure rate). If the images are technically adequate, the patient undergoes treadmill exercise stress, and then images are reacquired immediately, using special software to allow for the direct comparison of pre- and postexercise images. If pharmacologic stress testing with dobutamine is used, the doses of dobutamine are increased in a stepwise fashion and echocardiographic images are typically obtained each time the dose is increased. The safety of dobutamine stress echocardiography is comparable to that of a routine exercise stress test. Generally, SPECT is slightly more sensitive, and stress echo imaging is more specific for the diagnosis of CAD. Stress echocardiography may be preferred in some cases because some information is provided that is not obtained with radioisotopic scanning (ie, the presence of pericardial effusion, ventricular hypertrophy, or valve abnormalities); it also avoids exposure to radioactivity. The use of

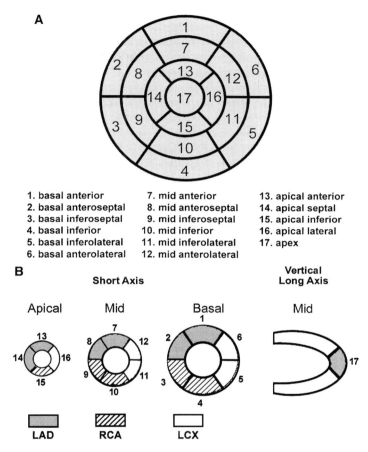

A

1. basal anterior
2. basal anteroseptal
3. basal inferoseptal
4. basal inferior
5. basal inferolateral
6. basal anterolateral

7. mid anterior
8. mid anteroseptal
9. mid inferoseptal
10. mid inferior
11. mid inferolateral
12. mid anterolateral

13. apical anterior
14. apical septal
15. apical inferior
16. apical lateral
17. apex

B

Short Axis

Vertical Long Axis

Apical   Mid   Basal   Mid

LAD   RCA   LCX

Fig. 2. (*A*) Left ventricular segmentation shows the standard nomenclature and segmentation used for SPECT myocardial perfusion imaging. The model divides the short-axis slices of the left ventricle into three major portions: apical, midventricular, and basal. The apex is a separate portion, which is analyzed from a vertical long-axis slice. The midventricular and basal short-axis slices are divided into six segments, whereas the apical short-axis slices are divided into four segments. The apex on the vertical long-axis slice represents one more segment. (*B*) Coronary artery territories. Although the anatomy of coronary arteries may vary substantially in individual patients, the location of myocardial perfusion abnormalities on SPECT or echocardiography imaging allows for a general prediction of which coronary artery is likely to be diseased. Shown here is the standardized assignment of coronary artery territories of the left anterior descending coronary artery (LAD), the right coronary artery (RCA), and the left circumflex coronary artery (LCX). The prediction of disease in the RCA and LCX is often less accurate because of substantial variation in extent to myocardial territories.

myocardial contrast echocardiography to add perfusion imaging to wall motion analysis is in development. Fig. 3 demonstrates the standard nomenclature for two-dimensional echocardiography; the coronary artery territory is the same as in Fig. 2B.

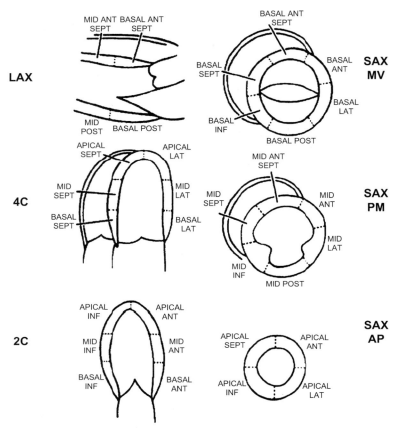

Fig. 3. Regional wall segments showing the left ventricle divided into 16 segments for two-dimensional echocardiography. These segments can be identified into a series of longitudinal views (LAX, 4C, 2C) or a series of short-axis views (SAM MV, SAX PM, SAX AP). The longitudinal and short-axis views overlap and complement each other. 2C, 2 chamber; 4C, 4 chamber; ANT, anterior; INF, inferior; LAT, lateral; LAX, long axis; POST, posterior; SAX AP, short-axis apex; SAX MV, short-axis mitral valve level; SAX PM, short-axis papillary muscle; SEPT, septum. (*From* Cerqueira MD, Weissman NJ, Dilsizian V, et al; for the American Heart Association Writing Group on Myocardial Segmentation and Registration for Cardiac Imaging. Standardized myocardial segmentation and nomenclature for tomographic imaging of the heart: a statement for healthcare professionals from the Cardiac Imaging Committee of the Council on Clinical Cardiology of the American Heart Association. Circulation 2002; 105(4):539–42; with permission.)

Pharmacologic stress testing

Patients who are unable to exercise because of physical limitations can be evaluated after receiving IV administration of dipyridamole, adenosine, or dobutamine in conjunction with the imaging modality. Dipyridamole and adenosine dilate all coronary vessels, increasing flow to all areas of the heart.

The enhanced dilation of normal coronary arteries, compared with that which occurs in significantly narrowed vessels, augments differences in flow that usually are not apparent at rest. These agents are suitable for use with radioisotopic imaging modalities that may readily demonstrate this flow heterogeneity. Because these agents affect flow but not heart rate or contractility, they are used only in conjunction with radioisotopic imaging but not with echocardiography. After the administration of dipyridamole or adenosine followed by either ^{201}Tl or ^{99m}Tc sestamibi (ie, the stress image), myocardial tissue supplied by a narrowed coronary artery typically demonstrates a perfusion defect that "fills in" during the rest image. Because of its short duration of action, adenosine is preferred to dipyridamole for this test. For a number of technical reasons, they remain the stress test of choice for patients who have LBBB.

Dobutamine is a β_1 agonist that, at IV high dosages (20 μg/kg/min to 40 μg/kg/min), increases myocardial contractility and heart rate in a manner and extent similar to exercise. Heart rate may not be affected to the same extent as contractility, and IV atropine is often administered to increase the heart rate to the maximal predicted heart rate for the patient's age. Dobutamine may be used in conjunction with either echocardiography or radioisotopic imaging for the diagnosis of CAD.

Mild side effects (nausea, flushing, and headache) are common with all of these agents and may occur in 75% of patients. Dipyridamole and adenosine can produce severe bronchospasm and should not be used in patients who have severe COPD. Adenosine causes chest pain in 50% of patients but has an exceedingly short half-life. Xanthine derivatives (eg, theophylline) and caffeine block adenosine receptors and should be avoided for 24 hours before a study. Dobutamine can increase arteriovenous (AV) nodal conduction and should not be used in patients who have atrial flutter and only carefully in patients who have atrial fibrillation. Adenosine can cause transient AV block.

Diagnostic use of exercise testing

A meta-analysis of 147 published studies has shown that the sensitivity and specificity of the exercise ECG for the detection of CAD (at least 50% stenosis angiographically) are 68% and 77%, respectively [17]. The sensitivity of the test increases with the severity of disease. The most common reasons for a false-positive exercise ECG are hypertension, cardiomyopathy, hyperventilation, and LVH.

The goal of the standard exercise treadmill test is to reach 90% of the maximal predicted heart rate for age (estimated as 220 per age). The electrocardiographic criteria for a positive test are considered to be a downward sloping or horizontal ST segment depression of more that 1 mm for three consecutive beats. The sensitivity and specificity for the diagnosis of CAD (70% occlusion in at least 1 vessel) are listed in Table 1 for the primary stress testing modalities. If stricter ECG criteria (ie, 2 mm ST depression) are used, the sensitivity decreases with increased specificity. False-positive stress tests occur more commonly in women, patients who have mitral valve prolapse, and baseline ST-T wave changes. Some experts suggest that all women should undergo imaging stress tests because of the problem of false-positive tests; the cost implication of that recommendation would be substantial, and the negative predictive value of the test remains high.

Stress test results predict prognosis as well. The factors that affect prognosis include the maximum amount of ST segment deviation during exercise, the presence or absence of angina, and the duration of exercise. The most extensive prognostic studies for abnormal stress tests have occurred in the field of radionuclide imaging, but the lessons carry over to treadmill and echo stress tests. The number, size, and location of abnormalities on stress myocardial perfusion studies reflect the location and extent of functionally significant coronary stenoses [18]. Echo and nuclear imaging can detect left ventricular dilation with stress, which suggests global, severe ischemia. Lung uptake of a radioactive tracer (^{201}Tl or ^{99m}Tc sestamibi) indicates stress-induced left ventricular dysfunction and suggests multivessel CAD. Many studies have shown that high-risk abnormal stress tests are associated with an increased risk of cardiac events. Importantly, normal echo and nuclear stress tests are highly predictive of a benign prognosis. In a review of 16 studies involving almost 4000 patients over 2 years, a negative perfusion scan was associated with a 0.9% rate of cardiac death per year, similar to the general population [19].

Positron emission tomography (PET) increases the scope of cardiac evaluation from perfusion and function to metabolic substrate use [20]. Whereas SPECT measures relative blood flow, PET can measure absolute blood flow. The sensitivity and specificity of PET are over 90% [21], but the cost effectiveness of the strategy is unknown. PET must be performed with vasodilator stress. Combined with CT angiography (described below), PET offers the possibility of a single test describing left ventricular size and function, coronary anatomy and baseline and stress-induced flow characteristics, and myocardial metabolism in the resting and stressed states. Research in this field is just beginning.

Advanced cardiac imaging: CT and MRI

CT is a highly sensitive technique for detecting coronary artery calcium, and its clinical usefulness is being evaluated [7]. ECG gating allows data acquisition within 1 to 2 breath holds, making it a fast test with limited radiation exposure. Calcium is easy to distinguish, and coronary calcium is highly sensitive for atherosclerotic CAD. The calcium score is an index of calcium deposition in multiple arterial segments and is a good approximation of the overall plaque burden in the coronary tree. High calcium scores are associated with an increased risk of myocardial infarction [22] and offers improved discrimination over conventional risk factors in the identification of people with CAD [23]. Whether calcium scores are useful in the initial diagnosis of patients who have angina pectoris is unclear. Coronary CT angiography is a new technique using multislice CT and IV contrast with fast ECG gating and specialized software to reconstruct the coronary arteries. This technique is presently being used mostly in research studies, but it is available for clinical use in patients who have chest discomfort and equivocal stress test results or for patients who refuse cardiac catheterization to define the extent of CAD. The safety and efficacy of CT angiography in the initial emergency department evaluation of patients who presented with chest pain has been demonstrated [24].

MR coronary angiography also is under development and can detect the major coronary vessels. High-speed MRI techniques allow for the simultaneous assessment of myocardial perfusion with MRI contrast agents [15]. MR perfusion imaging with dipyridamole [25] or dobutamine [26] as the stress agent compares favorably with SPECT and echocardiography in the diagnosis of CAD.

Coronary angiography and revascularization strategies

The 1999 ACC/AHA Guidelines for Coronary Angiography [27] outline the indications and contraindications for angiography. Class I indications for angiography include CCS class III or IV angina on medical treatment (angina at moderate exertion) and high-risk criteria on noninvasive testing, regardless of angina severity. High-risk stress tests are defined as more than 1 mm of ST segment depression, ischemia at a low workload (<5 METS), and ischemia involving a large territory of the LV myocardium. Class IIa recommendations include angina that improves with therapy but remains present; serial noninvasive testing showing progressively worsening abnormalities; patients who cannot tolerate medical therapy; patients who have angina who cannot be adequately risk stratified because of disability or illness; and individuals whose occupation involves the safety of others (pilots, bus drivers, and similar jobs) who have abnormal but not high-risk stress test results. There are no absolute contraindications to coronary arteriography. Relative contraindications include acute or chronic renal failure, active gastrointestinal bleeding, acute stroke, severe anemia, coagulopathy, unexplained fever or active untreated infection, severe uncontrolled hypertension, documented anaphylactoid reaction to angiographic contrast agents, and decompensated congestive heart failure. Renal insufficiency occurs in 0% to 5% of patients who do not have preexisting renal dysfunction and 10% to 40% of patients who have baseline renal insufficiency. Pretreatment with IV hydration (0.45% saline), N-acetylcysteine (600 mg twice daily), and limiting the use of IV contrast are the most effective means for mitigating renal dysfunction. In patients who are suspected of having iodine contrast allergy, pretreatment with corticosteroids and treatment with H_1 and H_2 histamine antagonists may reduce allergic complications. Major morbidity and mortality from coronary angiography is rare. In a survey of nearly 60,000 patients, the mortality from angiography was 0.11%; myocardial infarction occurred in 0.05% of patients; and stroke occurred in 0.07% of patients [28]. The most frequent major complication is vascular access complication (0.43%).

Coronary revascularization can be performed with either percutaneous coronary intervention (PCI) or coronary artery bypass surgery (CABG). Currently, 80% of PCI procedures in the United States are performed with a drug-eluting coronary stent coated with sirolimus or paclitaxel [29]. Revascularization should be considered in patients who have limiting angina despite medications or high-risk features on clinical history, stress testing, or catheterization. Patients who have multivessel CAD, proximal left anterior descending or left main CAD, reduced LV function, or a large ischemic burden as found by stress testing should be referred for revascularization. Five-year rates of MI and death are similar between PCI and CABG [30], although CABG generally yields more complete revascularization and more complete resolution of symptoms. Recent data favor CABG in high-risk patients who have reduced ejection fraction and diabetes [31]. The choice of drug-eluting stents over bare metal stents is associated with lower rates of restenosis, reduced angina, and fewer repeat revascularizations [32].

Prognosis

Coronary artery disease is a chronic condition; however, certain patients are at an increased risk for death and nonfatal myocardial infarction in the short term (1 year). The four characteristics that best predict risk are reduced left ventricular ejection fraction, the extent and severity of CAD, a recent plaque rupture event (STEMI or non-STEMI), and noncardiac comorbidity. The Coronary Artery Surgery Study (CASS) [33] is the largest dataset of patients who underwent medical treatment for symptomatic CAD. In that study, patients who were able to perform less than 4 METS of work on a treadmill and had significant ST segment depression had an annual mortality of greater than 5% per year [33]. Those who were able to exercise for 10 METS and had no ischemic ECG changes had an annual mortality of less than 1% per year. Patients who present at a younger age and those who do not alter modifiable risk factors may have more aggressive disease. Unfortunately, we do not have an adequate means to predict which plaque is likely to rupture and cause events. Therefore, the ability of a stress test to predict MI is reduced because many of the plaques that cause events are not flow limiting.

Medical treatment of angina pectoris

Medical management of angina pectoris falls into two categories: antianginal drugs [1,34,35], which may improve symptoms and exercise performance, and vasculoprotective agents [36–38], which modify the biology of atherosclerosis. A major advance in drug therapy has been the demonstration that long-acting antithrombotic agents and vigorous lipid-lowering therapy can improve outcomes in selected patients who have CAD. Angina that occurs with exercise usually is caused by an increase in myocardial oxygen demand that cannot be met because of a fixed arterial obstruction. A decrease in or cessation of the work that produced angina usually results in a prompt reduction in myocardial oxygen demand. Therefore, rest or a decrease in the level of activity may relieve angina in 1 to 2 minutes. If anxiety is a contributing or provoking factor, myocardial work may take longer to decrease, and the episode of angina may be prolonged. Antianginal medications reduce angina and prolong exercise time but have not been demonstrated to improve the rate of mortality [34].

Antianginal drugs

Nitrates

Traditionally, nitroglycerin has been an inexpensive mainstay of treatment of patients who have angina pectoris. Initially, these agents were believed to increase coronary blood flow by producing coronary artery dilation. Although nitrates may increase coronary blood flow in patients who have spasm or may increase collateral flow to obstructed vessels, evidence suggests that the mechanism of action of nitrates in most patients is not an increase in blood flow but a decrease in myocardial oxygen demand and peripheral vascular resistance. These compounds produce dilation of the venous circulation, resulting in reduced cardiac work and smaller left ventricular chamber size. Thus, the beneficial antianginal effect of nitrates is caused primarily by peripheral vasodilation.

Sublingual nitroglycerin is still the drug of choice for the relief and prevention of acute episodes of angina pectoris in most patients [29]. The initial dose should be small (0.4 mg) to minimize unpleasant side effects (flushing, headache, and light-headedness) in patients for whom higher dosages may be unnecessary. Patients should be taught that it is important that their pain be relieved as soon as possible, and they should be instructed to take nitroglycerin whenever such symptoms appear. Angina often produces discomfort and anxiety, which may increase heart rate and blood pressure and, hence, increased myocardial oxygen demand. If pain is not relieved by 2 to 3 tablets of nitroglycerin (the patient should wait for 3 minutes between doses) or if the use of nitroglycerin increases suddenly and dramatically, the patient should be instructed to call a physician or to go immediately to an emergency facility because of the danger of impending myocardial infarction. Nitroglycerin may lose potency on storage; patients should be advised not to keep tablets longer than 3 to 4 months after opening the bottle, and if pain is not relieved and usual side effects are not experienced.

Prophylactic use of nitroglycerin is of particular value in patients who have angina in response to specific and reproducible stress, despite other therapies. It is important to teach the patient to use sublingual nitroglycerin correctly. The patient should cease the activity that caused angina, take sublingual nitroglycerin, and sit down to avoid the possible untoward effects of hypotension (increased in the standing position). The most common side effects are flushing and headache, both of which may diminish with increasing usage of the drug. Constant serum levels of nitrate predispose to the development of tolerance [39]. It appears that a 12- to 14-hour nitrate-free interval is needed for the drug to exercise its maximal effect [40]. Therefore, patients who develop increasing angina while using the transdermal patch may benefit by changing to an oral nitrate regimen or by removing the patch at night [24]. The side effects of all long-acting nitrates are similar to those produced by sublingual nitrates. Many patients have already experienced the headaches produced by sublingual nitroglycerin before being treated with a long-acting preparation. Phosphodiesterase type 5 inhibitors (ie, sildenafil, vardenafil, and tadalafil) and nitrates should not be used within 24 hours of one another because of the potential for serious hypotension [29]. Nitrates may increase oxidative stress and induce paradoxical vasoconstriction [41].

β-Blockers

In many respects β blockade is an ideal approach to the treatment of angina. β-blockers reduce oxygen consumption by lowering heart rate, myocardial contractility, and systemic blood pressure. An added benefit for patients who have ischemic heart disease is that β blockade reduces the incidence of arrhythmias. The dosage of a β-blocker can be increased rapidly over hours or days until the desired effect is obtained. The heart rate is a useful guide to treatment; sinus bradycardia at a rate at rest between 50 and 60 beats per minute is a reasonable goal. However, the ideal dosage is one that not only results in mild sinus bradycardia at rest but also blocks an increase in heart rate with exercise. The dosage necessary to produce this effect and that necessary to relieve angina pectoris may vary considerably. Side effects of β-blockers have been overemphasized in recommending treatment of angina pectoris [42]. Erectile dysfunction occurs in 1% or less of the susceptible population. Asthma is still a relative contraindication, and selective β_1 antagonists should be used. Patients who have chronic obstructive pulmonary disease or peripheral vascular disease commonly have no difficulties tolerating β-blockers.

Calcium channel blockers

Calcium channel blockers (CCB) dilate coronary and systemic arteries, reducing oxygen consumption and increasing coronary blood flow. They are indicated in the treatment of both stable and unstable angina and are also effective antihypertensive agents. Although there was early concern about short-acting calcium channel blockers [43], recent trials demonstrate no increased morbidity or mortality in patients receiving long-acting CCBs [44,45] for hypertension. The CCBs approved by the US Food and Drug Administration for use in patients who have angina pectoris are amlodipine, diltiazem, nicardipine, long-acting nifedipine, and verapamil. The common side effects of the dihydropyridine calcium channel blockers (amlodipine, nicardipine, and nifedipine) are dizziness, flushing, headache, nausea, diarrhea, and, because of systemic vasodilation, peripheral edema. The major adverse effect is severe hypotension, which, in association with a reflex tachycardia, can actually intensify myocardial ischemia in some patients. Amlodipine is safe in patients who have left ventricular dysfunction. It only rarely affects AV conduction. Verapamil is prescribed more commonly for the treatment of hypertension or arrhythmias but is an effective antianginal. However, it has a more potent negative inotropic effect than other calcium channel blockers and significantly retards AV conduction. Therefore, it should not be used in patients who have compromised left ventricular function or with sinus bradycardia, sick sinus syndrome, or AV block. Diltiazem also significantly retards AV conduction, but it has less of a negative inotropic effect than verapamil and, in contrast to the dihydropyridines, is unlikely to cause hypotension or other vasodilatory side effects (eg, flushing, headache, edema).

Combination therapy

None of the antianginal classes has been demonstrated to be significantly better in head-to-head trials. Combination therapy is often an underused strategy [1,34]. Some combinations (eg, β-blockers plus verapamil or possibly diltiazem) should be avoided because of concern about bradycardia. There are no data on the combinations of all three classes. In the initial evaluation of patients who have angina, cardiac catheterization may be recommended before reaching this level (catheter guidelines).

Vasculoprotective drugs

General recommendations for patients who have angina pectoris include smoking cessation, blood pressure control, lipid modification, use of antiplatelet agents, and modifications to diet and exercise [1,36,37,46]. According to the recent recommendations of the Seventh Report of the Joint National Committee on Prevention, Detection, Evaluation, and Treatment of High Blood Pressure (JNC-7), blood pressure control is less than 130/80 mm Hg for high-risk patients in whom CAD is suspected. Exercise training [47], after safety is confirmed by provocative testing, is recommended for all patients who have angina pectoris. In one study [48], an exercise training program had better 1-year outcomes in major adverse cardiac events and exercise capacity compared with percutaneous intervention in patients who had single-vessel CAD. The American Heart Association step 2 diet [1] is recommended, but there are few data to support improved clinical outcomes. However, the Lyon Diet Heart Study [49] has demonstrated a 47% reduction in cardiac events in patients randomized to a Mediterranean diet compared with a Western diet with similar caloric intake. Efforts at weight control and smoking cessation are mandatory. A comprehensive risk factor modification strategy has been demonstrated to reduce major cardiac events in patients who have CAD [50] and in those with diabetes mellitus [51].

Antiplatelet agents

Aspirin remains the cheapest and arguably the most effective agent for reducing platelet aggregation. The AHA/ACC guidelines consider aspirin use to be a class 1 recommendation for patients who have angina. Unless there are proven significant contraindications, all patients who have angina should be receiving 81 mg to 150 mg of aspirin daily. Clopidogrel, an inhibitor of ADP-induced platelet aggregation, should be used in patients who are allergic to aspirin. The risks of antithrombotic therapy relate to the increased risk of bleeding or platelet dysfunction. Most of these drugs must be stopped several days before the patient undergoes elective surgical procedures.

Angiotensin-converting enzyme inhibitors

Angiotensin-converting enzyme (ACE) inhibitors should be used in patients who have angina who have a history of myocardial infarction, hypertension, left ventricular systolic dysfunction, or diabetes, as well as in patients who have impaired renal function and for whom their use is not contraindicated. However, many patients presenting for the first time with symptoms of angina may not have absolute indications for their use. The Heart Outcomes Prevention Evaluation (HOPE) trial [36] and European Trial on Reduction of Cardiac Events with Perindopril in Stable Coronary Artery Disease (EUROPA) [52] suggest that reduced cardiac events occurred in high-risk patients, but the routine use of ACE inhibitors in a lower risk cohort of patients who had CAD in the Prevention of Events with Angiotensin Converting Enzyme Inhibition (PEACE) trial [53] did not confirm those previous studies.

Statins

Statin use is associated with a 25% to 35% reduction in cardiac events and mortality and a 25% to 30% reduction in the need for coronary revascularization [54]. In the REVERSAL study [37], treatment for 18 months with atorvastatin, 80 mg, slowed the progression of CAD, measured by intravascular ultrasonography, compared with pravastatin, 40 mg. The

Treating to New Targets (TNT) trial [55] demonstrated a reduction in clinical events among patients who had stable coronary artery disease treated with atorvastatin, 80 mg (achieved mean LDL of 77 mg/dL) compared with atorvastatin, 10 mg daily. There was only a 1% increase in the risk of abnormalities in aminotransferase levels (1.2% versus 0.2%). The NCEP ATP-III recommends a target LDL cholesterol level of less than 100 mg/dL for all patients who have CAD, whereas for high-risk patients, an alternative treatment goal is an LDL cholesterol level of less than 70 mg/dL [56]. Whether patients who have angina pectoris without CAD should receive statins is unknown.

Other treatments for angina pectoris

For patients who have chronic angina pectoris despite maximal medical therapy and limited or no revascularization options, novel therapies, including enhanced external counter-pulsation [57], transmyocardial revascularization [58], and metabolic therapy with ranolozine [43] or trimetazidine [59], can be considered. A complete discussion of these options is outside the scope of this review.

Summary

Angina pectoris is a clinical manifestation of myocardial ischemia. Complete evaluation consists of a review of risk factors, a careful history, and, typically, a provocative test. Stress testing can be performed with exercise (treadmill, bicycle, or arm ergometry) or pharmacologic agents that increase cardiac work (dobutamine) or dilate the coronary vessels (adenosine or dipyridamole). Patients who have high-risk features found by clinical history or by stress testing should be referred for coronary angiography and possible revascularization. Comprehensive management of patients who have angina (with or without revascularization) includes smoking cessation, diet and weight control, vasculoprotective drugs (aspirin, statins, and possibly ACE inhibitors), and antianginal medications (nitrates, β-blockers, and calcium channel blockers). These strategies have led to an important reduction in morbidity and mortality over the past 2 decades, and the focus on implementing guidelines for patients who are currently undertreated is expected to improve outcomes further.

References

[1] Gibbons RJ, Abrams J, Chatterjee K, et al. ACC/AHA/ACP-ASIM guidelines for the management of patients with chronic stable angina: a report of the American College of Cardiology/American Heart Association Task Force on Practice Guidelines (Committee on Management of Patients With Chronic Stable Angina). J Am Coll Cardiol 1999;33(7): 2092–197.

[2] Grundy SM. Primary prevention of coronary heart disease: integrating risk assessment with intervention. Circulation 1999;100(9):988–98.

[3] Grundy SM. Coronary calcium as a risk factor: role in global risk assessment. J Am Coll Cardiol 2001;37(6):1512–5.

[4] Fuster V, Pearson TA, Co-Chairs. 27th Bethesda conference: matching the intensity of risk factor management with the hazard for coronary disease events. J Am Coll Cardiol 1996; 27(5):957–1047.

[5] National Cholesterol Education Program (NCEP) Expert Panel on High Blood Cholesterol. Detection, evaluation, and treatment of high blood cholesterol in adults: adult treatment panel III [third report]. Washington, DC: National Heart, Lung and Blood Institute; 2001. Bethesda (MD), NIH Publication #01–3670. Available at: http://www.nhlbi.nih.gov/guidelines/cholesterol/index.htm. Accessed January 3, 2006.

[6] Boden WE. High-density lipoprotein cholesterol as an independent risk factor in cardiovascular disease: assessing the data from Framingham to the Veterans Affairs high-density lipoprotein intervention trial. Am J Cardiol 2000;86(12, Suppl 1):19–22.

[7] O'Rourke RA, et al. American College of Cardiology/American Heart Association expert consensus document on electron-beam computed tomography for the diagnosis and prognosis of coronary artery disease. J Am Coll Cardiol 2000;36(1):326–40.

[8] Sandler G. The importance of the history in the medical clinic and the cost of unnecessary tests. Am Heart J 1980;100:980.

[9] Campeau L. Grading of angina pectoris [letter]. Circulation 1976;54(3):522–3.

[10] Zouridakis E, et al. Markers of inflammation and rapid coronary artery disease progression in patients with stable angina pectoris. Circulation 2004;110:1747–53.

[11] Kragelund C, et al. N-Terminal pro-B-type natriuretic peptide and long-term mortality in stable coronary heart disease. N Engl J Med 2005;352(7):666–75.

[12] Gibbons RJ, et al. ACC/AHA guidelines for exercise testing: a report of the American College of Cardiology/American Heart Association Task Force on Practice Guidelines (Committee on Exercise Testing). J Am Coll Cardiol 1997;30(1):260–311.

[13] Lee TH, Boucher CA. Noninvasive tests in patients with stable coronary artery disease. N Engl J Med 2001;344(24):1840–5.

[14] Hlatky M, Mark D. Economics and cardiovascular disease, in heart disease: a textbook of cardiovascular medicine. 6th edition. Philadelphia: WB Saunders; 2001. p. 19–26.

[15] Beller G. Relative merits of cardiovascular diagnostic techniques. In: Braunwald E, Zipes DP, Libby P, editors. Heart disease: a textbook of cardiovascular medicine. 6th edition. Philadelphia: WB Saunders; 2001. p. 422–41.

[16] Wackers F. SPECT detection of coronary artery disease. In: Narula VDaJ, editor. Atlas of nuclear cardiology. Philadelphia: Current Medicine; 2003. p. 63–77.

[17] Gianrossi R, Detrano R, Mulvihill D, et al. Exercise-induced ST depression in the diagnosis of coronary artery disease. A meta-analysis. Circulation 1989;80:87–98.

[18] Ritchie JL, et al. Guidelines for clinical use of cardiac radionuclide imaging: report of the American College of Cardiology/American Heart Association Task Force on Assessment of Diagnostic and Therapeutic Cardiovascular Procedures (Committee on Radionuclide Imaging), developed in collaboration with the American Society of Nuclear Cardiology. J Am Coll Cardiol 1995;25(2):521–47.

[19] Brown KA. Prognostic value of thallium-201 myocardial perfusion imaging: a diagnostic tool comes of age. Circulation 1991;83(2):363–81.

[20] Dilsizian V. SPECT and PET techniques. In: Narula VDaJ, editor. Atlas of nuclear cardiology. Philadelphia: Current Medicine; 2003. p. 19–46.

[21] Schelbert HR. Measurements of myocardial metabolism in patients with ischemic heart disease. Am J Cardiol 1998;82(Suppl 1):K61–7.

[22] Raggi P, et al. Identification of patients at increased risk of first unheralded acute myocardial infarction by electron-beam computed tomography. Circulation 2000;101(8):850–5.

[23] Guerci AD, et al. Comparison of electron beam computed tomography scanning and conventional risk factor assessment for the prediction of angiographic coronary artery disease. J Am Coll Cardiol 1998;32(3):673–9.

[24] White C, Kuo O, Kelemen MD, et al. Chest pain evaluation in the emergency room: can multi-detector CT provide a comprehensive evaluation? AJR Am J Roentgenol 2005;185:533–40.

[25] Mathejssen N, et al. Comparison of ultrafast dipyridamole magnetic resonance imaging with dipyridamole sestamibi SPECT for detection of perfusion abnormalities in patients with one-vessel coronary artery disease: assessment by quantitative model fitting. Magn Reson Med 1996;35:221.

[26] Nagel E, et al. Noninvasive diagnosis of ischemia-induced wall motion abnormalities with the use of high-dose dobutamine stress MRI: comparison with dobutamine stress echocardiography. Circulation 1999;99:763.

[27] Scanlon PJ, et al. ACC/AHA guidelines for coronary angiography: a report of the American College of Cardiology/American Heart Association Task Force on practice guidelines (Committee on Coronary Angiography), developed in collaboration with the Society for Cardiac Angiography and Interventions. J Am Coll Cardiol 1999;33(6):1756–824.

[28] Noto TJ Jr, et al. Cardiac catheterization 1990: a report of the Registry of the Society for Cardiac Angiography and Interventions. Cathet Cardiovasc Diagn 1991;24(2):75–83.

[29] Abrams J. Chronic stable angina. N Engl J Med 2005;352(24):2524–33.

[30] Hoffman SN, et al. A meta-analysis of randomized controlled trials comparing coronary artery bypass graft with percutaneous transluminal coronary angioplasty: one- to eight-year outcomes. J Am Coll Cardiol 2003;41(8):1293–304.

[31] Hannan EL, et al. Long-term outcomes of coronary-artery bypass grafting versus stent implantation. N Engl J Med 2005;352(21):2174–83.

[32] Al Suwaidi J, et al. Impact of coronary artery stents on mortality and nonfatal myocardial infarction: meta-analysis of randomized trials comparing a strategy of routine stenting with that of balloon angioplasty. Am Heart J 2004;147:815–22.

[33] Weiner DA, Ryan TJ, McCabe CH, et al. Prognostic importance of a clinical profile and exercise test in medically treated patients with coronary artery disease. J Am Coll Cardiol 1984; 3:772–9.

[34] Thadani U. Treatment of stable angina. Curr Opin Cardiol 1999;14:349–58.

[35] Heidenreich PA, et al. Meta-analysis of trials comparing [beta]-blockers, calcium antagonists, and nitrates for stable angina. JAMA 1999;281(20):1927–36.

[36] Heart Outcomes Prevention Evaluation Study Investigators. Effects of an angiotensin-converting-enzyme inhibitor, ramipril, on cardiovascular events in high-risk patients. N Engl J Med 2000;342(3):145–53.

[37] Nissen SE, et al. Effect of intensive compared with moderate lipid-lowering therapy on progression of coronary atherosclerosis: a randomized controlled trial. JAMA 2004;291(9): 1071–80.

[38] Cannon CP, et al. Intensive versus moderate lipid lowering with statins after acute coronary syndromes. N Engl J Med 2004;350(15):1495–504.

[39] Gori T, Parker J. The puzzle of nitrate tolerance: pieces smaller than we thought? Circulation 2002;106:2404–8.

[40] Gori T, Parker J. Nitrate tolerance: a unifying hypothesis. Circulation 2002;106:2510–3.

[41] Munzel T, et al. Evidence for enhanced vascular superoxide anion production in nitrate tolerance: a novel mechanism underlying tolerance and cross-tolerance. J Clin Invest 1995;95: 187–94.

[42] Ko DT, et al. [beta]-Blocker therapy and symptoms of depression, fatigue, and sexual dysfunction. JAMA 2002;288(3):351–7.

[43] Chaitman BR, et al. Anti-ischemic effects and long-term survival during ranolazine monotherapy in patients with chronic severe angina. J Am Coll Cardiol 2004;43(8): 1375–82.

[44] Blood Pressure Lowering Treatment Trialists. Effects of different blood-pressure-lowering regimens on major cardiovascular events: results of prospectively-designed overviews of randomised trials. Lancet 2003;362(9395):1527–35.

[45] The ALLHAT Officers and Coordinators for the ALLHAT Collaborative Research Group. Major Outcomes in high-risk hypertensive patients randomized to angiotensin-converting enzyme inhibitor or calcium channel blocker vs diuretic: the Antihypertensive and Lipid-Lowering Treatment to Prevent Heart Attack trial (ALLHAT). JAMA 2002;288(23): 2981–97.

[46] Heart Protection Study Collaborative. MRC/BHF Heart Protection Study of cholesterol lowering with simvastatin in 20,536 high-risk individuals: a randomised placebo controlled trial. Lancet 2002;360(9326):7–22.

[47] Gielen S, Schuler G, Hambrecht R. Exercise training in coronary artery disease and coronary vasomotion. Circulation 2001;103(1):1–6.

[48] Hambrecht R, et al. Percutaneous coronary angioplasty compared with exercise training in patients with stable coronary artery disease: a randomized trial. Circulation 2004;109(11): 1371–8.

[49] de Lorgeril M, et al. Mediterranean diet, traditional risk factors, and the rate of cardiovascular complications after myocardial infarction: final report of the Lyon Diet Heart Study. Circulation 1999;99(6):779–85.

[50] Haskell W, et al. Effects of intensive multiple risk factor reduction on coronary atherosclerosis and clinical cardiac events in men and women with coronary artery disease: the Stanford Coronary Risk Intervention Project (SCRIP). Circulation 1994;89(3):975–90.

[51] Gaede P, et al. Multifactorial intervention and cardiovascular disease in patients with type 2 diabetes. N Engl J Med 2003;348(5):383–93.

[52] Fox KM, for the EURopean trial On reduction of cardiac events with Perindopril in stable coronary Artery disease Investigators. Efficacy of perindopril in reduction of cardiovascular events among patients with stable coronary artery disease: randomised, double-blind, placebo-controlled, multicentre trial (the EUROPA study). Lancet 2003;362(9386):782–8.

[53] The PEACE Trial Investigators. Angiotensin-converting-enzyme inhibition in stable coronary artery disease. N Engl J Med 2004;351(20):2058–68.

[54] Group SSS. Randomised trial of cholesterol lowering in 4444 patients with coronary heart disease: the Scandinavian Simvastatin Study Group. Lancet 1994;344:1383–9.

[55] LaRosa JC, et al. Intensive lipid lowering with atorvastatin in patients with stable coronary disease. N Engl J Med 2005;352(14):1425–35.

[56] Grundy SM, et al. Implications of recent clinical trials for the National Cholesterol Education Program Adult Treatment Panel III guidelines. J Am Coll Cardiol 2004;44(3):720–32.

[57] Michaels AD, et al. Two-year outcomes after enhanced external counterpulsation for stable angina pectoris (from the International EECP Patient Registry [IEPR]). Am J Cardiol 2004; 93(4):461–4.

[58] Bridges CR, et al. The Society of Thoracic Surgeons practice guideline series: transmyocardial laser revascularization. Ann Thorac Surg 2004;77(4):1494–502.

[59] Marzilli M, Klein W. Efficacy and tolerability of trimetazadine in stable angina: a meta-analysis of randomized, double-blind, controlled trials. Coron Artery Dis 2003;14:171–9.

ELSEVIER
SAUNDERS

THE MEDICAL
CLINICS
OF NORTH AMERICA

Med Clin N Am 90 (2006) 417–438

Arrhythmias in the Office

Luis H. Haro, MD[a],*, Erik P. Hess, MD[b], Wyatt W. Decker, MD[a]

[a]*Department of Emergency Medicine, Mayo Clinic College of Medicine, Rochester, MN, USA*
[b]*Division of Critical Care, Department of Medicine, Mayo Clinic, Rochester, MN, USA*

The incidence of patients who present to the office with arrhythmia and hemodynamic instability is unknown. Emergency medical systems data, based on ambulance runs, are available only for patients who have had a cardiac arrest. When faced with an unstable or potentially unstable patient, however, we must be prepared to act quickly, safely, and accurately. This following text addresses the general approach to such a patient; provides necessary information on office emergency preparation, including training, rapid response team protocol, and the use of automated external defibrillators; and addresses the identification and initial office management of the various rhythms that are capable of threatening a patient's life.

Preparing for office emergencies

Being prepared to deal with an emergency in the office setting is not an easy task. It requires protocols, equipment, and training, all of which take considerable effort and time. The current recommended level of preparedness is not clear from the literature. Brief reports in the literature demonstrate the variability in equipment and training [1,2]. In 1984, a survey of office physicians reported that 11% had adequate equipment to manage common office emergencies. Seventy-nine percent were basic cardiac life support (BCLS)-certified, 35% were advanced cardiac life support (ACLS)-certified, 19% had defibrillators, 35% had intravenous (IV) catheters, and 40% had laryngoscopes. Only 42% of the participants responded to the questionnaire [1].

Training may be the most important effort that leads to office preparedness. Investigators from Department of Pediatrics at Duke University

---

* Department of Emergency Medicine, Mayo Clinic, 200 First Street, Rochester, MN 55905.

E-mail address: luis.haro@mayo.edu (L.H. Haro).

School of Medicine conducted a prospective, randomized, controlled trial of primary care practices (pediatric, family practice, and health departments) that evaluated the effectiveness of an office-based educational program [2]. This program was designed to improve the preparation of primary care practices for pediatric emergencies. Practices that agreed to participate were assigned randomly to the intervention or the control group. Unannounced mock codes were conducted in the intervention practices. Practices were expected to respond to the mock code using their own staff, equipment, and local emergency medical system. After the exercise, there was a structured debriefing session. The primary outcome measures were obtained by survey 3 to 6 months after intervention and included (1) purchase of new pediatric emergency equipment and medications, (2) receipt or updating of basic life support/pediatric advanced life support/advanced life support training by staff members, and (3) development of written emergency pediatric protocols. The control practices received no interventions during the trial and completed a similar outcome survey. Thirty-nine practices (20 intervention, 19 control) completed the trial. Intervention practices were more likely to develop written office protocols (60% versus 21%) and receive additional basic and advanced life support training 3 to 6 months after the intervention (118 versus 54). There were no significant differences in the purchase of new equipment or medications.

Literature that is specific to arrhythmias in the office setting is scarce. Ultimately, an arrhythmia that presents with concerning complaints (Box 1)

Box 1. Symptomatic arrhythmias: warning symptoms of hemodynamic compromise

Symptoms
- Lightheaded
- Chest pressure/pain
- Dyspnea
- Palpitations
- Orthostatic symptoms
- Syncope
- Cardiopulmonary arrest

Signs
- Hypotension
- Heart rate >130 beats/min (bpm) or <50 bpm
- Temperature <35°C
- Cyanosis
- Cool extremities
- Altered mental status
- Tachypnea

needs to be managed in an emergency department (ED) with ACLS measures. Response times of ambulances vary, but they can be up to 25 minutes [3–6]. Response times from an internally affiliated emergency team might be faster. Hence, the focus of this discussion is based on providing the tools to assess and manage a patient for the first 30 minutes in the office setting.

The most important step for all patients who present with an arrhythmia or with any life-threatening presentation is being prepared for a cardiopulmonary arrest. Preparedness requires basic cardiac life support training, a simple office emergency protocol, some basic equipment, and rapid access to an emergency response team.

Education

The author recommends training all office personnel in basic life support and the use of an automated external defibrillator (AED). This training is easily obtainable from the American Heart Association (available at http://www.americanheart.org. The basic life support health care provider course teaches cardiopulmonary resuscitation (CPR) skills for helping victims of all ages, and the use of an AED. It is intended for health care providers, such as physicians, nurses, respiratory therapists, physical and occupational therapists, physician's assistants, aides, medical or nursing assistants, and other allied health personnel. The course length is 6 to 8 hours. Education is the first step in setting up your office protocol for emergencies.

Equipment

Many commercially prepared first aid kits are available for the office setting. They range from first aid kits (eg, Rescue One First AID) to ACLS rescue kits similar to code carts (eg, Banyan Stat Kit). Each office practice should make its own assessment of needs. Prices range from $130 to $995. In addition to the kit, a separate key component is an AED or conventional defibrillator for practices that manage adults who are at risk. Retrospective chart review data demonstrate that dialysis centers have the highest relative incidence of cardiac arrest (0.746 per practice annually), followed closely by cardiology, internal medicine, family medicine, and urgent care centers (0.01 per practice annually). All other medical and dental practices have a low incidence (≤ 0.002 per practice annually) [7,8].

Basic office emergency protocol

Form a rapid response team

It is vital to have an identified team within your office staff that responds to internal emergencies. A "code" is a rapid response signal that brings help to the patient, irrespective of the severity of the patient's status. It is used commonly in in-hospital settings and ranges from help for a hypoglycemic event, syncope, or allergic reaction to a cardiopulmonary arrest. A good rule is to "overtriage" and call a code before making a full assessment. This approach maintains the code team skills, brings immediate help to the patient, and most importantly, prevents further deterioration of the patient's status.

Establish response team responsibilities

Responsibilities of the response team include:

- Calling for help (911 or the emergency response team for your institution). Have a code team member identified who will have this responsibility.
- Relocating the patient, if possible. Ideally a two- or three-member team allows for a rapid transfer of the patient to an area within the office that has a first aid kit, an oxygen tank, and an AED. If this is impossible because of logistics, have a small cart that can be brought to the patient.
- Incorporating a family member to the team. If the patient's ability to provide a history is impaired, family members can provide valuable information; often do not get in the way of the team; and most importantly, are intimately aware of the status of the patient, the efforts that are being made to help, and are not surprised as easily when poor outcomes result [9–11].
- Providing basic life support (BLS), if necessary. A brief summary of BLS and the use of an AED are described later in this article.
- Debriefing. After a rapid response team is activated it is critical to learn from the experience and to prepare for future events as best as possible.

General approach to the patient with a witnessed collapse in the office setting

Check the victim for a response. If there is a response (the victim answers or moves), check the level of alertness, chief complaint, blood pressure, pulse, and oxygenation; if a significant abnormality is present, ask any staff member to call for help. Office practices that are not adjacent to a hospital or without established efficient emergency protocols should call 911 immediately. After the emergency medical systems are activated, move the patient to an examination room, ask for the first aid kit or its equivalent, and address abnormal vital signs systematically before moving on (eg, if hypoxic, administer oxygen supplementation; if hypotensive, keep the patient supine and establish an IV with a 250- to 500-mL fluid bolus in 15 minutes if possible). Blood glucose also should be checked early on in the evaluation of the patient. If hypoglycemia is present, provide glucose. A gel is available in most kits if the patient cannot swallow. If an IV is established, provide 1 ampule of D50 (50% dextrose). If no IV is available, 1 to 2 mg of intramuscular Glucagon can be administered, which increases serum glucose levels reliably. Get a targeted history and physical, if possible, and reassess the patient frequently until help arrives. Significant changes in the pulse that suggest a potential lethal arrhythmia are discussed in further detail later in this article.

If the victim does not respond, shout for help, send someone for help, or if on your own, consider leaving the victim and going for help, or calling 911 or a code team immediately. It is important to remember a major principle of emergency medicine, never create a second victim: the rescuer. Take precautions for infectious disease—use mouth masks and gloves. Return to the patient and open the airway by tilting the head and lifting the chin (Fig. 1). Keeping the airway open, look, listen, and feel for breathing (more than an occasional gasp). Look for chest movements and listen at the victim's mouth for breath sounds. Feel for air on your cheek (Fig. 2).

If the patient is breathing (other than an occasional gasp), place him/her in the recovery position (on his/her side). The airway of an unconscious victim who is breathing spontaneously is at risk of obstruction by the tongue and from aspiration of mucus and vomit. Placing the victim on his/her side helps to prevent these problems and allows fluid to drain from the mouth. Check for continued breathing.

If the victim is not breathing, do a head tilt and chin lift. Use barrier device precautions—pocket face masks (preferably with a one-way valve) or a bag valve and an oropharyngeal airway should be immediately available; insert it and begin ventilations. Give two effective rescue breaths, each of which makes the chest rise and fall. If there is difficulty achieving an effective breath, recheck the victim's mouth and remove any obstruction. Recheck that there is adequate head tilt and chin lift. Make up to five attempts to achieve two effective breaths. Even if unsuccessful, move on to assessment of circulation.

Assess the patient for signs of circulation. This includes looking for any movement, including swallowing or breathing, and checking if the carotid pulse is present. Check the pulse for at least 10 seconds; if there is a pulse, continue rescue breathing, if necessary, until the victim starts to breathe on his/her own. About every minute, recheck for signs of circulation; take no more than 10 seconds each time. If the victim starts to breathe on his/her own but remains unconscious, place the victim in the recovery position. Check the victim's condition and be ready to turn the victim onto his/her back and restart rescue breathing if breathing stops.

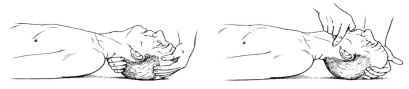

Fig. 1. Rescue breathing head tilt and remove foreign body or dentures if present. (Courtesy of the Mayo Clinic, Rochester, MN; with permission.)

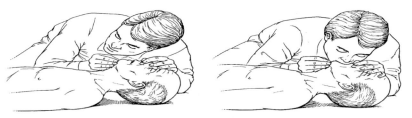

Fig 2. Look for a chest rise, listen, and feel for air. If patient is not breathing, provide two slow breaths; in the office setting, the use of a barrier device is highly recommended. (Courtesy of the Mayo Clinic, Rochester, MN; with permission.)

If there are no signs of circulation or if you are at all unsure, start chest compression. After 15 compressions, tilt the head, lift the chin, and give two effective breaths; continue compressions and breaths in a ratio of 15:2 until help arrives (Fig. 3).

The tachycardias

Ventricular fibrillation and ventricular tachycardia

Usually, ventricular tachycardia (VT) and ventricular fibrillation (VF) are caused by acute coronary syndromes that lead to ischemic areas of myocardium. Other nonischemic causes are evolution from stable to unstable VT, and untreated premature ventricular complexes with R-on-T phenomenon. Multiple drugs, or electrolyte or acid–base abnormalities can prolong the relative refractory period and cause VT or VF. Finally, primary or secondary QT prolongation are well-known reasons for the development of these arrhythmias. Initially, the goal is to resuscitate the patient by focusing on the airway, breathing, and circulation and performing rapid defibrillation. Box 2 describes the ECG criteria of VF and pulseless VT. Figs. 4 and 5 provide rhythm strips on both.

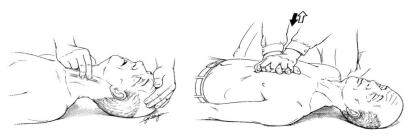

Fig. 3. Assess pulse, if absent begin CPR. (Courtesy of the Mayo Clinic, Rochester, MN; with permission.)

Box 2. Ventricular fibrillation/pulseless ventricular tachycardia

Ventricular fibrillation
- **Rate/QRS complex:** unable to determine; no recognizable P, QRS, or T waves
- **Rhythm:** indeterminate; pattern of sharp up (peak) and down (trough) deflections
- **Amplitude:** measured from peak-to-trough; often used subjectively to describe VF as fine (peak-to-trough 2 to <5 mm), medium-moderate (5 to <10 mm), coarse (10 to <15 mm), very coarse (>15 mm)

Ventricular tachycardia
- **Note ≥3 consecutive premature ventricular complexes (PVCs):** ventricular tachycardia
- **Rate:** ventricular rate >100 bpm; typically 120–250 bpm
- **Rhythm:** no atrial activity seen, only regular ventricular
- **PR:** nonexistent
- **P waves:** seldom seen but present; VT is a form of AV dissociation (which is a defining characteristic for wide-complex tachycardias of ventricular origin versus supraventricular tachycardias with aberrant conduction)
- **QRS complex:** wide and bizarre, "PVC-like" >0.12 s, with large T wave of opposite polarity from QRS

Automated external defibrillators

The importance of early defibrillation in the treatment of sudden cardiac death cannot be overstated. American Heart Association guidelines seek to ensure that a defibrillator reaches the victim at the earliest appropriate opportunity; hence, the rationale for phoning first or calling a "code" that brings a defibrillator to the patient's side. This is to ensure that the health care staff does not become so consumed with providing CPR that it persists far too long before summoning the emergency system. Therefore, the initial call for help in the office after assessing unresponsiveness should result in

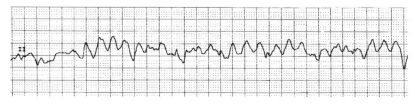

Fig. 4. Ventricular fibrillation. (Courtesy of the Mayo Clinic, Rochester, MN; with permission.)

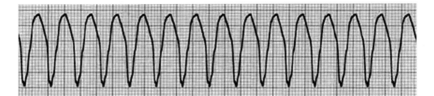

Fig. 5. Ventricular tachycardia. (Courtesy of the Mayo Clinic, Rochester, MN; with permission.)

someone arriving with a defibrillator—in any of its forms—in-hospital code response team, outpatient clinic on-site emergency code cart, or out-of-hospital emergency medical services (EMS) unit.

An AED is a device that incorporates a rhythm–analysis system and a shock-advisory system for victims of cardiac arrest. The AED advises a shock, and the operator must take the final action to deliver the shock. The International Guidelines for Cardiopulmonary Resuscitation and Emergency Cardiovascular Care [12] conclude that early CPR is the best treatment for cardiac arrest until the arrival of an AED and advanced cardiac life support care. Early CPR can prevent ventricular fibrillation from deteriorating to asystole, may increase the chance of successful defibrillation, and contributes to the preservation of heart and brain function. For victims of sudden cardiac arrest that is due to VF or pulseless VT, the single greatest determinant of survival is the time from collapse to defibrillation. A survival rate as high as 90%—among victims of witnessed VF cardiac arrest—has been reported when defibrillation is achieved within the first minute of collapse. These survival rates for out of hospital cardiac arrest have been reported in cardiac rehabilitation programs that were equipped with defibrillators. Survival rates decline 7% to 10% with every minute that defibrillation is delayed, such that a victim of cardiac arrest without defibrillation beyond 12 minutes has only a 2% to 5% chance of survival [12].

The most important reason to use an AED is its ease, because there is no need to learn what a shockable rhythm looks like, no need to adjust Joules or worry about a monophasic or biphasic mode. Additionally, most AEDs remind you to continue CPR if the rhythm is not shockable.

Operating an automated external defibrillator.
1. Power on.
2. Attach electrode pads.
3. Press "Analyze."
4. State "Clear" and press shock if so advised.

Do this up to three times if advised. Repeat cycles of three shocks and 1 minute of CPR until "no shock indicated" message is displayed. After "no shock indicated" messages, check pulse. If no pulse, perform CPR for 1 minute and analyze again. Continue same cycle until help arrives.

Although these steps are followed with all AEDs, there are variations in models that change how the steps are performed. Because of this, it is important to train staff on the specific model that they will be using.

Maintaining an automated external defibrillator. Maintaining AEDs appropriately is vital to ensure a continuous state of readiness. Most malfunctions in AEDs are due to improper maintenance or battery failure. To limit potential problems, manufacturers have developed AEDs that perform automatic self-testing, which saves time, improves testing consistency, and minimizes unnecessary battery expenditure. Battery options now include a rechargeable lead acid battery and a high-capacity, extended shelf-life lithium sulfate battery that needs no recharging and no maintenance. Maintenance checklists provide for a standardized inspection and should be used to ensure that the AEDs are kept in a state of readiness. Inspections and checklists help to identify and prevent deficiencies by providing a uniform way to inspect devices, and by increasing the user's familiarity with the equipment.

AEDs are part of the basic life support course for health care providers; they allow for nonphysician staff to deliver the most important life saving measure without having to interpret a rhythm. In the author's opinion, all office-based practices that see adult patients who are at risk for sudden cardiac death should have one readily available.

Conventional/defibrillator/monitor. If an AED is not available and a conventional/defibrillator/monitor is, then:

1. Power on monitor and defibrillator (could require one or two controls).
2. Attach three-lead monitor cable, display rhythm through quick-look sternal-apex paddles.
3. Assess for a shockable rhythm by viewing monitor display (there should be no CPR or other patient manipulation during rhythm assessment).
4. Charge to 200 J, 300 J, or 360 J monophasic or clinically equivalent biphasic for shocks 1, 2, and 3.
5. Shock ("Clear!") up to three times if a shockable rhythm is present, following the same assess, charge, and shock sequence.

After three shocks or after any non-VF/VT rhythm on monitor, check pulse. If no pulse, perform CPR for 1 minute and analyze again. Continue same cycle until help arrives.

Tachycardias with a pulse

If a patient has a pulse, measure blood pressure and assess the cardiac rhythm and rate. Common tachycardias that are encountered in an office-based setting and are capable of producing hemodynamic instability include supraventricular tachycardia (SVT), atrial fibrillation (AF), and atrial flutter.

Paroxysmal supraventricular tachycardia

In paroxysmal SVT (PSVT) there is a reentry phenomenon where impulses arise and recycle repeatedly in the atrioventricular (AV) node because of areas of unidirectional block in the Purkinje fibers. Frequently, there also is an accessory conduction pathway in most healthy people in whom many factors can provoke the paroxysm (eg, caffeine, hypoxia, cigarettes, stress, anxiety, sleep deprivation, numerous medications). PSVT occurs with an increased frequency in patients who have chronic obstructive pulmonary disease, coronary artery disease, or congestive heart failure. Usually, the clinical manifestations are palpitations that are felt by the patient at the onset. Other symptoms include lightheadedness, anxiety, and an otherwise uncomfortable feeling. They also can experience poor exercise tolerance with high ventricular rates (150–180 bpm). Syncope, altered mental status, and cardiac arrest are uncommon. When a patient loses a pulse and has this organized rhythm by definition, it is labeled a pulseless electrical activity, which is a rare event. Box 3 describes the ECG criteria, and Fig. 6 demonstrates a sample rhythm strip.

When a patient presents to the office with these symptoms and PSVT is recognized, an attempt at a therapeutic/diagnostic maneuver with vagal stimulation is reasonable. Some patients will have experience with specific maneuvers that have been useful for them and some will have tried it before seeking care. Therefore, it is important to review briefly the past medical history, medications, and experience with vagal maneuvers. If this has not been performed and the patient is stable, it is reasonable to attempt such an intervention. Waxman and colleagues [13] showed that carotid massage and the Valsalva maneuver (VM) are the most powerful physical maneuver for termination of PSVT, and it has a significant vagal effect on AV node conduction. In their study, maneuvers that reflexly increase vagal tone were used to terminate the tachycardia in 68 consecutive patients who had PSVT. Fifty-seven episodes were terminated with carotid sinus massage (CSM), 5 were terminated with VMs, and 6 were terminated pharmacologically with phenylephrine. Luber and colleagues [14], in a retrospective chart

---

Box 3. Supraventricular tachycardia: defining ECG features

- **Rate:** exceeds upper limit of sinus tachycardia (>120 bpm); seldom <150 bpm; up to 250 bpm
- **Rhythm:** regular
- **PR:** seldom seen because rapid rate causes P wave loss in preceding T waves or because the origin is low in the atrium
- **QRS complex:** normal, narrow (usually 0.10 s)

Key: regular, narrow-complex tachycardia without P waves.

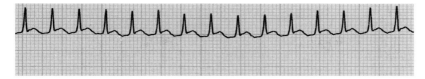

Fig. 6. Supraventricular tachycardia. (Courtesy of the Mayo Clinic, Rochester, MN; with permission.)

review of 111 patients who presented to the ED with PSVT, reported that 26 patients (23%) spontaneously converted to having a normal sinus rhythm (NSR) without therapy while waiting. In 44 patients who received vagal maneuvers, 22 had successful conversion. The rest had pharmacologic conversion (41 of 48 patients with adenosine). Overall, 71% of patients were discharged from the ED. Only 4% had a recurrence of their SVT after discharge.

There is debate on what maneuver should be attempted first. Lim and colleagues [15] conducted a prospective, randomized study of CSM versus VM for PSVT in the ED in 148 patients. The VM converted PSVT to NSR in 19% of the cases, whereas CSM converted PSVT to NSR in 10% of cases. A combination of both had an overall success rate of 27.7%. CSM is performed gently, yet firmly, for 2 minutes to abort the episode. In patients with a history of carotid artery disease or who are at risk for a stroke, a VM or other maneuvers are preferable. If these maneuvers are unsuccessful, administration of adenosine, 6 mg IV for adults, is a reasonable option, although this therapy is contraindicated in patients who have asthma or reactive airway disease and in patients with heart rates above 200 bpm, because of the possibility of degeneration into a ventricular tachycardia (when the blocking capabilities of the AV node are inhibited). Management of these patients is done best in an emergency setting. Occasionally, patients who have hemodynamic instability from PSVT require direct current (DC) cardioversion, which can be performed by paramedics at arrival or by trained physicians.

Atrial fibrillation and atrial flutter with rapid ventricular response

The hallmark of these arrhythmias is atrial impulses that run faster than the sinus node impulses. In AF, impulses take multiple, chaotic, random pathways through the atria. Atrial flutter is characterized by impulses that take a circular course around the atria and set up the flutter waves. The mechanism of impulse formation is a reentry pathway that leads to tachycardia.

Patients who present with new-onset AF need an evaluation for the underlying cause as well as management of the arrhythmia. Etiologies of AF include conditions that distend or irritate the musculature of the atria, such as cardiac ischemia, congestive heart failure, valvular heart disease, cardiomyopathies, and recent cardiac surgery. Pulmonary etiologies, such as chronic obstructive pulmonary disease, pulmonary embolism, and pulmonary hypertension, also can cause AF. Systemic etiologies, including hyperthyroidism and medication use, should be considered. There is a subset of patients in whom the work-up for an underlying cause is unrevealing, and lone AF is diagnosed [16]. Table 1 describes the ECG criteria for AF and atrial flutter. Figs. 7 and 8 are examples of these rhythms.

Signs and symptoms are functions of the rate of ventricular response to atrial fibrillatory waves. AF with rapid ventricular response (RVR) symptoms are mostly due to a loss of "atrial kick" that may lead to a decrease in cardiac output and decreased coronary perfusion; patients often complain of dyspnea at rest or on exertion. Other patients perceive the irregular rhythm as "palpitations" and even can be asymptomatic, especially at rest. Other presenting symptoms include chest pain or discomfort, fatigue, or lightheadedness.

There are four essential question to ask when faced with a patient who has a fibrillation/flutter and an RVR:

1. Is the patient clinically unstable? (Does the patient have ischemic chest pain? Is the patient hypotensive?)
2. Is the cardiac function impaired? (Does the patient have a known depressed left ventricular function?)
3. Is Wolff-Parkinson-White syndrome (WPW) present? (Is there a history of WPW, and are earlier ECGs available for comparison?)
4. Have the symptoms been present for less than 48 hours or longer than 48 hours?

Table 1
Atrial fibrillation and flutter

Fibrillation	Flutter
Rate: wide ranging ventricular response to atrial rate of 300–400 bpm	• Atrial rate 220–350 bpm • Ventricular response is a function of AV node block or conduction of atrial impulses • Ventricular response rarely >150–180 bpm because of AV node conduction limits
Rhythm: classic "irregularly irregular"	• Regular • Set ratio to atrial rhythm (eg, 2:1 or 3:1)
P waves: chaotic atrial fibrillatory waves	• No true P waves seen • Flutter waves in "sawtooth" pattern
PR interval: cannot be measured	• Cannot be measured
QRS: remains δ .10–.12 s unless QRS complex distorted by fibrillation/flutter waves or by conduction defects through ventricles	

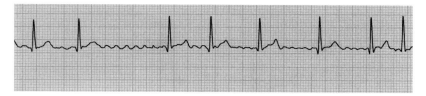

Fig. 7. Atrial fibrillation. (Courtesy of the Mayo Clinic, Rochester, MN; with permission.)

Is the patient unstable?

One must treat unstable patients urgently; call 911, administer oxygen, place the patient in the supine position, and obtain a blood pressure. If hypotension is present, an IV should be placed. In addition, have someone obtain the office AED or a conventional monitor/defibrillator. While resuscitative efforts get underway, attempt to get a targeted history. If an AED is available, power on, analyze, and if advised to shock, clear everyone and do so. AF or flutter are not perceived by the AED as a shockable rhythm; furthermore, the AED does not measure or interpret other physiologic parameters. In this scenario, one can wait for EMS to arrive or if AF or flutter with RVR is suspected, switch to a conventional defibrillator/monitor. After an IV is established and an RVR is confirmed (usually >150 bpm), power on the defibrillator, set on synchronize, place the energy at 100 J, clear all staff, deliver a shock, and verify response. If no response, increase subsequently to 150 J, 200 J, 300 J, and 360 J. Usually, after the first or second attempt the patient converts to a sinus tachycardia or NSR. In the infrequent event that the patient loses a pulse, start CPR and provide support as described in the pulseless rhythm section of this article.

Is cardiac function impaired?

If a patient does not have hypotension but is experiencing significant chest pain/pressure or dyspnea, provide 325 mg aspirin, establish IV access, provide a 250-mL bolus, and simultaneously review the patient's medications. If help has not arrived, control the heart rate. This can be achieved effectively by administering metoprolol; a reasonable starting dose is 5 mg IV. Diltiazem is an excellent alternative and is one of the most frequently used in the ED, mostly because of the lack of frequent contraindications

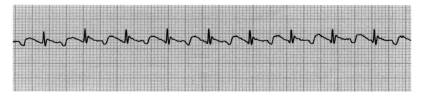

Fig. 8. Atrial flutter. (Courtesy of the Mayo Clinic, Rochester, MN; with permission.)

that are associated with β-blockers and the high rate of success with a first dose. A ventricular rate of less than 130 bpm is ideal; however, this should not be the target in the office setting because hypotension after drug administration is not uncommon. Obviously, this scenario is handled best in the ED. Finally, if a patient develops severe chest pain or has significant ST segment abnormalities, it is not unreasonable to perform synchronized cardioversion while awaiting transport, especially if the patient has had symptoms for less than 48 hours. If the patient exhibits signs of congestive heart failure or has known poor left ventricular function, synchronized cardioversion or amiodarone is the best therapeutic intervention.

Is Wolff-Parkinson-White syndrome present?

AF or flutter in combination with WPW (Fig. 9) deserves special mention because of the potential for development of an unstable tachycardia if treated inappropriately. Patients who have AF and WPW should not receive conventional rate control with β-blockers, calcium channel blockers, digoxin, or adenosine because of the potential inhibition of the AV node that might be inhibiting chaotic atrial rates. If this AV node is inhibited, the potential for a reentry of an atrial impulse through an accessory pathway increases dramatically, and VT or VF might result.

Have symptoms been present for less that 48 hours?

In the stable patient who has minimal complaints and an RVR (usually <130 bpm), administration of a β-blocker or calcium channel blocker is preferable if available. There is no urgency to intervene in this case; patients can be referred by ambulance to the ED where further management will be performed.

Young patients who have normal or near normal hearts and a history of recurrent paroxysmal AF (PAF) have been treated in Italy with a "pill in the pocket approach" [17]. This approach is reserved for patients who have converted in the hospital or the ED with a single dose of oral propafenone or flecainide with success and without side effects (78% of all patients who had PAF). This out-of-hospital self-administration was done after the onset

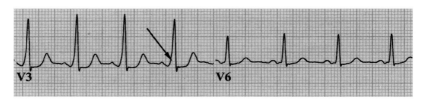

Fig. 9. Wolff-Parkinson-White syndrome: normal sinus rhythm with delta wave (*arrow*) notching of positive upstroke of QRS complex. (Courtesy of the Mayo Clinic, Rochester, MN; with permission.)

of heart palpitations in 210 patients (mean age $\pm$ SD, 59 $\pm$ 11 years). During a mean follow-up of 15 $\pm$ 5 months, 165 patients (79%) had a total of 618 episodes of arrhythmia; of those episodes, 569 (92%) were treated 36 $\pm$ 93 minutes after the onset of symptoms. Treatment was successful in 534 episodes (94%); the time to resolution of symptoms was 113 $\pm$ 84 minutes. Among the 165 patients who had recurrences, the drug was effective during all of the arrhythmic episodes in 139 patients (84%). Adverse effects were reported during one or more arrhythmic episodes by 12 patients (7%), including atrial flutter at a rapid ventricular rate in 1 patient and "noncardiac" side effects in 11 patients. The numbers of monthly visits to the ED and hospitalizations were significantly lower during follow-up than during the year before the target episode ($P < .001$ for both comparisons). The investigators concluded that in a selected, risk-stratified population of patients who had recurrent AF, pill-in-the-pocket treatment is feasible and safe, with a high rate of compliance by patients, a low rate of adverse events, and a marked reduction in ED visits and hospital admissions. No study in the United States has evaluated such an approach.

Other infrequent tachycardias, such as multifocal atrial tachycardia and junctional tachycardia, are the result of emphysema, cardiomyopathy, asthma, or pulmonary hypertension. Usually, they are managed by controlling the underlying exacerbation of the primary disease and not the actual arrhythmia (eg, management with β-agonists of asthma or emphysema and not the arrhythmia) [12].

The bradycardias

Bradycardia is a common finding during the clinical evaluation of healthy and ill patients; its exact incidence is unknown. It is found commonly in two settings. Often, bradycardia is detected incidentally in the asymptomatic patient during a routine history and physical examination that is performed during an office visit. A rhythm strip or ECG that is obtained for other purposes may bring the bradycardia to the physician's attention. Additionally, bradycardia may be detected in the symptomatic patient. Often, symptoms and signs are nonspecific and include dizziness, fatigue, weakness, or shortness of breath; however, symptoms can present dramatically with syncope, hypotension, or a depressed level of consciousness. Establishing a correlation between signs and symptoms and simultaneous rhythm abnormalities or a change in rhythm is key to diagnosis [18]. The following discussion highlights ways to identify specific types of bradycardias, including sinus bradycardia, AV block, junctional rhythm (Fig. 12), and idioventricular rhythm (Fig. 13). Even bradycardias that typically portend a benign prognosis can produce profound signs and symptoms that should be managed more aggressively [19].

There are many potential etiologies to consider in the bradycardic patient, both intrinsic and extrinsic. Acutely, it important to consider life-threatening and potentially treatable causes, before proceeding with a

Box 4. Causes of bradycardia

Life-threatening
- Myocardial ischemia
- Electrolyte imbalance
  - Hyperkalemia
  - Hypokalemia
- Medication toxicity
  - β-Blocker
  - Calcium channel blocker
  - Digoxin
- Sick sinus syndrome

Other[a]

Intrinsic
- Idiopathic degeneration (aging)
- Infiltrative diseases
  - Amyloidosis
  - Sarcoidosis
  - Hemochromatosis
- Collagen vascular diseases
  - Systemic lupus erythematosus
  - Scleroderma
  - Rheumatoid arthritis
- Myotonic muscular dystrophy
- Surgical trauma
  - Valve replacement
  - Correction of congenital heart disease
  - Heart transplantation
- Infectious diseases
  - Lyme disease
  - Chagas disease
  - Endocarditis

Extrinsic
- Autonomically-mediated syndromes
  - Neurocardiogenic syncope
  - Carotid-sinus hypersensitivity
  - Situational disturbances
    - Coughing
    - Micturition
    - Defecation
    - Vomiting

- Drugs
  - Antiarrhythmic agents
  - Clonidine
- Hypothyroidism
- Hypothermia
- Neurologic disorders

---

[a] *Adapted from* Mangrum JM, DiMarco JP. The evaluation and management of bradycardia. N Engl J Med 2000;342(10):705.

more comprehensive evaluation (Box 4). Causes to consider immediately include myocardial ischemia or infarction, electrolyte imbalance, medication toxicity, or sick sinus syndrome. If any of these etiologies is suspected, transport to the nearest ED should be considered strongly. A crucial electrolyte imbalance to consider is hyperkalemia, especially in a patient who has known renal failure [20]. If hyperkalemia is a suspected cause in a patient who has profound bradycardia, obtaining confirmation with ECG, administering albuterol by metered dose inhaler or nebulizer, establishing IV access, and treating the patient with calcium chloride and sodium bicarbonate before transport to the nearest ED can be life saving. Additional medication effects to consider include β-blocker, calcium channel blocker, or digoxin toxicity. Box 4 also highlights other causes of bradycardia to consider after the emergency has been handled and the patient is in the hospital or returns to the office for follow up.

As outlined in the ACLS algorithm for bradycardia, management depends on the severity of the patient's symptoms and the nature of the arrhythmia. For patients who have significant signs and symptoms that are due to the bradycardia, such as depressed consciousness or hypotension, immediate treatment is indicated. Atropine is the recommended initial pharmacologic intervention before transport to the nearest ED. If the patient fails to respond to atropine, transcutaneous pacing is appropriate. In the patient who does not have significant signs and symptoms and in whom the bradycardia was discovered incidentally, management depends on the propensity of the bradycardia to degenerate to complete heart block. In Mobitz type II second-degree AV block (Fig. 10) and third-degree heart block (Fig. 11), the bradycardia is likely to progress; permanent transvenous pacing may be indicated, even in the asymptomatic patient. Placement of pacing electrodes in preparation for transcutaneous pacing before transport to the ED is appropriate [12]. In patients who have more benign bradycardias without significant signs and symptoms, continued elective evaluation in the office setting is appropriate. This can include sinus bradycardia and first-degree AV block. ECG criteria for common bradycardias that are encountered in the outpatient setting are described in Box 5.

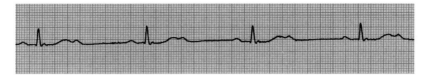

Fig. 10. Mobitz II second-degree heart block. (Courtesy of the Mayo Clinic, Rochester, MN; with permission.)

Transfer considerations

Before consideration of transfer, initial efforts should focus on stabilizing the patient as described above. It should be recognized early in the process that the unstable patient is best cared for in a hospital-based setting that is equipped to handle the full extent of a life-threatening emergency. After it becomes clear that a patient may have a life-threatening condition (including most sustained arrhythmias), arrangements should be made to transfer. Two important principles in the transfer of patients include stabilizing the patient's condition before transfer and arranging for an appropriate mode of transport.

Stabilizing the patient's condition before transfer

All available resources should be used to initiate resuscitation of a patient. This can include the use of an AED, placement of a peripheral line, and administration of oxygen (in some settings ventilating with a bag-valve mask or even endotracheal intubation may be needed). The extent of the resuscitation depends on the available equipment and personnel. It is important for the office practice to be aware of the ACLS algorithms and be prepared to initiate steps should a patient present in an unstable fashion.

Appropriate mode of transport

When a patient is transported to another facility, it is a time of potential vulnerability. Therefore, the provider must arrange for a level of transport that is equipped to care for the patient's presenting complaints and any likely complications or deteriorations [21]. Usual options to the office practice include

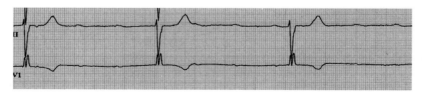

Fig. 11. Complete heart block. (Courtesy of the Mayo Clinic, Rochester, MN; with permission.)

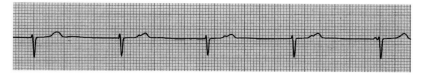

Fig. 12. Junctional rhythm. (Courtesy of the Mayo Clinic, Rochester, MN; with permission.)

private automobile with the patient driving, private automobile with a family member or companion driving, basic life support (capable of CPR), and advanced life support (capable of providing ACLS level of care). It may be appropriate to consider helicopter transport when longer transports with a high level of care are necessary. The mode of transport often is looked at simply as a mechanism to transport the patient to a hospital. Sometimes overlooked is the ability of a skilled paramedic to provide life-saving care. Because of this a patient who has unstable vital signs, including hypotension (systolic blood pressure less than 90 mm Hg), tachy- or bradyarrhythmias, or ongoing chest pain, generally should be transferred by ACLS-capable providers. These include emergency medical team (EMT) paramedics and flight nurses. Patients who have the above conditions are not ideal candidates for BLS or private automobile transports because—even if they are feeling well—they may deteriorate in route. Patients who may be able to be transported by private automobile (although they should not drive) include the healthy patient in whom a nonlife-threatening arrhythmia has resolved. Whenever there is doubt, it is in the patient's interest to err on the side of caution and to provide the highest level of transport that is available.

Much concern has focused on Emergency Medical Treatment and Active Labor Act (EMTALA) regulations surrounding transfers. The EMTALA was enacted in 1986 as part of the consolidated Omnibus Reconciliation Act of 1985, in response to concerns that some EDs were refusing to treat uninsured patients or were transferring them inappropriately to other facilities [22]. Since its inception, the law has expanded in scope and has had varying interpretations [23]. Although the legislation offers some helpful tips about the transfer of patients, it does not apply to patients who are cared for in the office/outpatient setting. A potential exception to that may be a clinic practice that is on hospital grounds and meets the definition

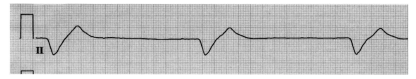

Fig. 13. Idioventricular rhythm. (Courtesy of the Mayo Clinic, Rochester, MN; with permission.)

Box 5. Bradycardia ECG criteria

Non–life-threatening
- **Sinus bradycardia**: sinus rhythm with a heart rate ≤60 bpm
- **First-degree AV block**: prolonged PR interval (>200 ms)
- **Second-degree AV block**: Mobitz type I (progressively lengthening PR interval until the P wave is not followed by a QRS complex)

Life-threatening
- **Mobitz type II**: nonconducted P wave with a constant PR interval before and after the nonconducted beats (see Fig. 10)
- **Third-degree AV block**: complete failure of AV nodal conduction with P waves completely dissociated from the QRS complexes (see Fig. 11)
- **Junctional rhythm**: slow regular rhythm with QRS complexes <120 ms. Rate is usually 40–60 bpm. Retrograde P waves may or may not be present. Typically is an escape mechanism during high-grade AV block (see Fig. 12).
- **Idioventricular rhythm**: slow regular rhythm with QRS complexes >120 ms. Rate is usually 30–40 bpm. P waves, if present, bear no relation to QRS complexes. Also an escape mechanism during high-grade AV block (see Fig. 13).

---

of a "dedicated ED." This is a facility that is licensed by the state as an ED and is held out to the public as a place that provides care for emergency medical conditions, and cares for patients on an urgent basis without a previously scheduled appointment. In this setting, the key elements of transferring are described in the EMTALA (Box 6). Compliance with these basic

---

Box 6. Emergency Medical Treatment and Active Labor Act transfer requirements

- Transferring facility provides medical treatment within its capacity to minimize risk of transfer to the patient.
- An accepting physician has been contacted at the receiving hospital and has agreed to treat the patient.
- The receiving hospital has space and qualified personnel available to treat the individual.
- Copies of medical records related to the reason for transfer are sent with the patient.
- Transfer is effected through qualified personnel and equipment as required, including appropriate life support measures.

tenants represents good patient care and professionalism. It is particularly important to contact the receiving facility to be sure that there is an accepting physician, and to send the patient with all appropriate documentation of testing and care that has been rendered.

References

[1] Kobernik MS. Management of emergencies in the medical office. Emerg Med 1986;4(1): 71–4.
[2] Bordley WC, Travers D, Scanlon P, et al. Office preparedness for pediatric emergencies: a randomized, controlled trial of an office-based training program. Pediatrics 2003;112(2): 291–5.
[3] Sempowski IP, Brison RJ. Dealing with office emergencies. Stepwise approach for family physicians. Can Fam Physician 2002;48:1464–72.
[4] Ota FS, Muramatsu RS, Yoshida BH, et al. GPS computer navigators to shorten EMS response and transport times. Am J Emerg Med 2001;19(3):204–5.
[5] Breen N, Woods J, Bury G, et al. A national census of ambulance response times to emergency calls in Ireland. J Accid Emerg Med 2000;17(6):392–5.
[6] Stiell IG, Wells GA, Field BJ, et al. Improved out-of-hospital cardiac arrest survival through the inexpensive optimization of an existing defibrillation program: OPALS study phase II. Ontario Prehospital Advanced Life Support. JAMA 1999;281(13):1175–81.
[7] Becker L, Eisenberg M, Fahrenbruch C, et al. Cardiac arrest in medical and dental practices: implications for automated external defibrillators. Arch Intern Med 2001;161(12):1509–12.
[8] Showan AM, Sestito JA. Organization of personnel and resources for airway management in the hospital and office environment. Crit Care Clin 2000;16(3):527–39.
[9] Clark AP, Aldridge MD, Guzzetta CE, et al. Family presence during cardiopulmonary resuscitation. Crit Care Nurs Clin North Am 2005;17(1):23–32.
[10] MacLean SL, Guzzetta CE, White C, et al. Family presence during cardiopulmonary resuscitation and invasive procedures: practices of critical care and emergency nurses. Am J Crit Care 2003;12(3):246–57.
[11] Meyers TA, Eichhorn DJ, Guzzetta CE. Do families want to be present during CPR? A retrospective survey. J Emerg Nurs 1998;24(5):400–5.
[12] Guidelines 2000 for Cardiopulmonary Resuscitation and Emergency Cardiovascular Care. Part 6: advanced cardiovascular life support: 7D: the tachycardia algorithms. The American Heart Association in collaboration with the International Liaison Committee on Resuscitation. Circulation 2000;102:I86.
[13] Waxman MB, Wald RW, Sharma AD, et al. Vagal techniques for termination of paroxysmal supraventricular tachycardia. Am J Cardiol 1980;46:655–64.
[14] Luber S, Brady WJ, Joyce T, et al. Paroxysmal supraventricular tachycardia: outcome after ED care. Am J Emerg Med 2001;19(1):40–2.
[15] Lim SH, Anantharaman V, Teo WS, et al. Comparison of treatment of supraventricular tachycardia by Valsalva maneuver and carotid sinus massage. Ann Emerg Med 1998; 31(1):30–5.
[16] Page RL. Newly diagnosed atrial fibrillation. N Engl J Med 2004;351:2408–16.
[17] Alboni P, Botto GL, Baldi N, et al. Outpatient treatment of recent-onset atrial fibrillation with the "pill-in-the-pocket" approach. N Engl J Med 2004;351(23):2384–91.
[18] Mangrum JM, DiMarco JP. The evaluation and management of bradycardia. N Engl J Med 2000;342(10):703–9.
[19] Gregoratos G, Abrams J, Epstein AE, et al. ACC/AHA/NASPE 2002 guideline update for implantation of cardiac pacemakers and antiarrhythmia devices: summary article. A report of the American College of Cardiology/American Heart Association task force on practice guidelines. Circulation 2002;106:2145.

[20] Zimmers T, Patel H. Cases in electrocardiograhy. Am J Emerg Med 2002;20(4):340–3.
[21] Roush WR. Principles of EMS systems. 2nd edition. Dallas (TX): American College of Emergency Physicians; McGraw-Hill Companies; 1994.
[22] General Accounting Office. Emergency care: EMTALA implementation and enforcement issues [#GAO-01-747]. Washington DC: General Accounting Office; 2001.
[23] Wanerman R. The EMTALA paradox. Ann Emerg Med 2002;40(5):464–9.

ELSEVIER
SAUNDERS

THE MEDICAL
CLINICS
OF NORTH AMERICA

Med Clin N Am 90 (2006) 439–451

Hypertensive Emergency and Severe Hypertension: What to Treat, Who to Treat, and How to Treat

John S. Flanigan, MD[a],*, David Vitberg, MD[b]

[a]Division of Emergency Medicine, University of Maryland School of Medicine,
Baltimore, MD, USA
[b]Combined Program of Internal Medicine and Emergency Medicine,
University of Maryland School of Medicine, Baltimore, MD, USA

Hypertensive emergency is a clinical syndrome of rapidly progressive end-organ damage associated with a significant elevation of blood pressure. The immediate reduction of blood pressure using potent intravenous (IV) agents is indicated to reduce the mortality rate, which ranges historically as high as 90%. Virtually all episodes of hypertensive emergency are associated with a diastolic blood pressure (DBP) >120 mm Hg; however, most patients who present with severe hypertension do not have a hypertensive emergency. It is crucial to recognize that not only will these patients not benefit from aggressive normalization of blood pressure but also there can be substantial morbidity caused by overly rapid decreases in blood pressure in patients who do not have rapidly evolving end-organ damage. Distinguishing between these two groups of patients is the first step in the safe management of significantly hypertensive patients. A thorough history, physical examination, and assessment of readily available laboratory tests will efficiently identify the minority of patients who need intensive treatment. Unfortunately, unclear terminology for clinically describing these patients is often a source of confusion and can present a barrier to correct management. As medical therapy grows more powerful, the attendant risks also grow in consequence. Definitions that served in the past now need refinement, based on the available evidence of the benefits and risks of therapy.

* Corresponding author. Division of Emergency Medicine, University of Maryland School of Medicine, 419 West Redwood Street, Suite 280, Baltimore, MD 21201.
 E-mail address: flanigirg@aol.com (J.S. Flanigan).

0025-7125/06/$ - see front matter © 2006 Elsevier Inc. All rights reserved.
doi:10.1016/j.mcna.2005.11.008

Definitions

Hypertensive crisis is traditionally defined as an elevation of diastolic blood pressure > 120 mm Hg. This category includes patients who have hypertensive emergency, hypertensive urgency, and severe hypertension. The term "crisis" suggests a need for immediate intervention, which is often contraindicated in these latter groups. For this reason, the use of this term should be de-emphasized.

Hypertensive emergency is defined by acute and rapidly evolving end-organ damage associated with significant hypertension, usually a DBP > 120 mm Hg. Controlling blood pressure within hours is desirable and requires admission to a critical care setting.

Hypertensive urgency is defined as a DBP > 120 mm Hg that requires improvement in blood pressure control over a period of 24 to 48 hours. This definition is problematic because, in the absence of evolving end-organ damage, there is little evidence of clinical benefit with the control of blood pressure over this period. Often the urgency is more in the mind of the treating physician than in the body of the patient. There are certainly occasions when improved short-term blood pressure control is needed, such as the imminent need for a procedure under anesthesia, but the clinician must carefully weigh the benefits of blood pressure control against the known risks of achieving it. Hypertensive urgency as a general descriptive term poses many of the same drawbacks as hypertensive crisis and therefore likewise should be de-emphasized.

Severe hypertension is defined usually as systolic blood pressure (SBP) > 180 mm Hg or DBP > 110 mm Hg, with some variability from study to study. The key definition of severe hypertension is the lack of rapidly evolving end-organ damage and a concomitant indication to gradually control the blood pressure.

The Joint National Committee (JNC) on Prevention, Detection, Evaluation, and Treatment of High Blood Pressure [1,2] has changed the classification of hypertension between the sixth and seventh report (Table 1).

Table 1
Changes in Joint National Committee classification of hypertension

JNC report no. [Ref. no.] and stages	SBP/DBP range (mm Hg)
JNC VI [1]	
High normal	130–139/85–89
Stage 1	140–153/90–99
Stage 2	160–179/100–109
Stage 3	180+/110+
JNC VII [2]	
Prehypertension	120–139/80–89
Stage 1	140–159/90–99
Stage 2	160+/100+

Malignant hypertension is an older term no longer in wide usage. It referred originally to elevated pressure associated with group IV Keith-Wagener-Barker retinopathy, papilledema, retinal hemorrhages and exudates, and is sometimes used to describe hypertensive emergency associated with central nervous system findings. Accelerated hypertension is another older term applied originally to hypertension associated with group III Keith-Wagener-Barker retinopathy and retinal hemorrhages and exudates. It has since been demonstrated that the Keith-Wagener-Barker classification of retinopathy does not accurately assess the severity of hypertension [3] or the clinical outcome [4,5], and these terms are no longer considered useful.

Demographics of hypertension and hypertensive emergency

According to the JNC VII [2], hypertension is the most common primary diagnosis in the United States (35 million office visits per year) affecting almost 25% of the population. Thirty percent of the population is unaware they have hypertension, and control rates for patients known to have hypertension still fall short of 50%. The consequences of hypertension are well described in JNC VII:

- In persons older than 50 years of age, systolic blood pressure greater than 140 mm Hg is a much more important cardiovascular disease (CVD) risk factor than diastolic blood pressure.
- The risk of CVD beginning at 115/75 mm Hg doubles with each increment of 20/10 mm Hg.

These demographics and the consequences of hypertension are well outlined in this report [2] and throughout the medical literature. In marked contrast, the prevalence and incidence of hypertensive emergency, crisis, and urgency are far from clear. There are several reasons for this, and reviewing them introduces the reader to the complexities of managing these conditions.

First, the lack of a consistent definition of hypertension extremes has resulted in variable data collection in published studies, making comparisons difficult. Second, much of the literature on hypertensive crisis and associated conditions is older. Although hypertension management is far from perfect now, there have been tremendous strides during the last 4 decades, and much of the cited literature is now 2 to 4 decades old. Third, hypertensive emergency is a heterogeneous condition probably resulting from a tiny percentage of poorly controlled essential hypertensive cases and even rarer cases of secondary hypertension. The acquisition of meaningful statistics describing such uncommon occurrences is problematic and susceptible to multiple biases such as enrollment in primary health care, socioeconomic status of the population, and referral bias in tertiary care centers. With these caveats in mind, the interpretation of the widely quoted incidence of hypertensive crisis of 1% of all hypertensive cases would suggest that as many as 500,000 Americans present for evaluation yearly, giving weight to the importance of correct diagnosis and management of this condition [6].

Pathophysiology of hypertensive emergency

The striking rapidity of end-organ damage and severity of blood pressure elevation at the time of presentation of hypertensive emergency are attributed to the failure of the normal autoregulatory function and to abrupt increases in systemic vascular resistance. There is concurrent endovascular injury, with fibrinoid necrosis of arterioles. The ensuing cycle of ischemia, platelet deposition, and further failure of autoregulation caused by the release of vasoactive substances accelerates the patient's clinical deterioration [7,8].

The specific triggers for this dramatic process usually are unknown and may well vary among the heterogeneous causes of the underlying hypertensive process. In any event, the bedside management of the patient is addressed usually to mitigating damage to whichever organ system is manifesting the most disease, rather than to modifying the underlying autoregulatory function.

Under normal conditions, tissue perfusion in the brain, heart, and kidneys remains relatively constant, despite normal fluctuations in blood pressure. In the presence of severe hypertension, this ability to autoregulate shifts upward to protect the exposed organ from excessive pressure. In both the normal situation and when upwardly shifted, the lower threshold of autoregulation (the threshold for hypoperfusion) is approximately 20% to 25% lower than the prevailing blood pressure [8]. This physiologic observation has been translated into a clinical recommendation to limit the initial lowering of blood pressure to 20% below pretreatment values.

Conditions associated with extremes of hypertension

Severe hypertension is seen disproportionately in association with secondary hypertension, and many causes of secondary hypertension are known to result in blood pressure lability, further disposing toward hypertensive crisis. Box 1 lists some of these conditions.

Although these conditions can underlie a hypertensive crisis, given the relative prevalence of essential hypertension, it is not surprising that this diagnosis accounts for most presentations of severe hypertension and hypertensive emergency. Many asymptomatic patients who have severe hypertension are unaware of their condition; however, most patients who experience a hypertensive emergency are aware of their condition [9] and have a history of inadequate treatment or of abrupt medication withdrawal. Centrally acting agents such as clonidine are often implicated in medication withdrawal, but rapid end-organ damage can result from the abrupt discontinuation of any potent regimen, and patients on high doses and multiple drug regimens need to understand the importance of avoiding the sudden discontinuation of medications.

Box 1. Causes of secondary hypertension

Neurologic conditions
- Autonomic hyperactivity (spinal cord injury, Guillain-Barré syndrome, and other causes)
- Baroreflex failure
- Cardiovascular accident
- Head trauma

Hormonal conditions
- Pheochromocytoma
- Renin- or aldosterone-secreting tumors

Pregnancy-associated conditions
- Eclampsia
- Preeclampsia

Immune conditions
- Scleroderma and other collagen vascular disease
- Vasculitis

Renal conditions
- Parenchymal renal disease, such as glomerulonephritis
- Renovascular disease

Drug-related conditions
- Drug interaction (eg, interactions of monamine oxidase inhibitor with tyramine, tricyclics, or sympathomimetics)
- Sympathomimetics (eg, cocaine, amphetamine, and phencyclidine)

Drug withdrawal conditions
- Abrupt discontinuation of antihypertensive medications
- Alcohol withdrawal

The role of chronic, progressive hypertension as a cause of hypertensive emergency is hard to specify in an age of widespread hypertension screening and treatment. Most patients are identified and at least partially treated well below the threshold for hypertensive emergency. Messerli [10] reviews the case of former President Franklin D. Roosevelt, with further editorial observations by Calhoun and Oparil [11], which throws light on the threshold for hypertensive emergency in chronically hypertensive patients and on the possible role played by secondary causes of hypertension in the extremes of hypertension. When hypertension was regarded medically as an "essential" adaptation to underlying vascular disease, President Roosevelt developed hypertension in his 50s, and within 10 years, he died of cerebral hemorrhage, with a final blood pressure of 300 mm Hg systolic and 190 mm Hg diastolic. Fig. 1 shows the time course of Roosevelt's hypertension.

Masserli [10] indicates that this 10-year time course is atypically rapid for essential hypertension, because the age of onset was late and the progression to death was relatively swift. As summarized by Calhoun and Oparil [11] in the associated editorial, the onset of essential hypertension in the fourth decade of life with an untreated survival of 20 years was more typical in the pretreatment era. This observation suggests that the long duration of asymptomatic severe hypertension, whether essential or secondary, before hypertensive disease manifests as hypertensive emergency.

Recognizing hypertensive emergency

Significant elevation of blood pressure is a common thread in the diagnosis of hypertensive emergency, but the key symptomatic manifestations of the syndrome vary widely, depending on the target organ involvement. The major target organs in hypertensive emergency are the brain, heart and great vessels, kidney, and the gravid uterus. One recent study by Zampaglione and colleagues [9] found single-organ involvement in 83%, two-organ involvement in 14%, and three or more organ involvement in only 3% of hypertensive emergencies. The relative frequency of end-organ involvement in hypertensive emergency is summarized in Table 2.

The initial assessment of hypertensive crisis is straightforward. A history and physical examination rapidly direct further investigation to the involved

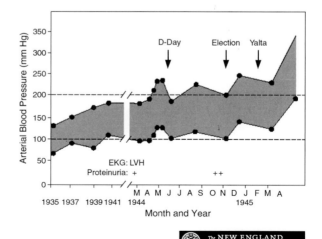

Fig. 1. Diastolic and systolic arterial pressure of Franklin D. Roosevelt from 1935 until his death on April 12, 1945. LVH, left ventricular hypertrophy. Data are from the diary of Dr. Howard G. Bruenn. (*From* Messerli FH. This day 50 years ago. N Engl J Med 1995;332:1038–9. © 1995 Massachusetts Medical Society; with permission.)

Table 2
Types of end-organ damage associated with hypertensive emergency

End-organ damage type	Cases (%)
Cerebral infarction	24.5
Intracerebral or subarachnoid bleed	4.5
Hypertensive encephalopathy	16.3
Acute pulmonary edema	22.5
Acute congestive heart failure	14.3
Acute myocardial infarction or unstable angina	12.0
Aortic dissection	2.0
Eclampasia	2.0

Data from Zampaglione B, Pascale C, Marchisio M, et al. Hypertensive urgencies and emergencies. Prevalence and clinical presentation. Hypertension 1996;27:144–7.

organs. Appropriate chemistry measurements and EKG are available widely. Urine toxicology for cocaine metabolites is helpful in select populations. Plain chest radiographs are useful for assessing volume status and cardiac size and are a first screen for aortic dissection. In patients whose condition is highly suspicious for aortic dissection (those who experience severe or ripping chest or abdominal pain, especially radiating to the back), further diagnostic studies with CT scanning of the chest with contrast is warranted. Unfortunately, renal function is often marginal and carefully balancing risks and benefits is called for. It bears repeating that aortic dissection accounted for only 2% of hypertensive emergencies in the above-cited series. With this in mind, CT screening for dissection in the emergent setting is not indicated routinely. This careful balancing of risk and benefit is not an issue concerning head CT for patients who display neurologic symptoms because these scans are performed initially without contrast, usually after the first control of blood pressure is achieved.

Overview of treatment of hypertensive emergency

After developing a high index of clinical suspicion of rapidly evolving end-organ damage, the clinician needs to initiate therapy in a timely fashion, keeping in mind the following:

- Promptly initiate goal-directed pharmacologic therapy with readily available agents, often before the diagnostic workup is completed.
- Ensure that the involved critical staff is familiar with dose ranges, infusion techniques, blood pressure monitoring requirements, and side effects of the medications used.
- Be mindful of practical considerations influencing the choice of pharmacologic therapy, including the need to transport the patient to multiple locations (emergency department, diagnostic radiology, operating room, catheterization lab, and intensive care unit). It is often difficult to maintain continuous IV infusions and even more difficult to maintain continuous intra-arterial pressure monitoring during this process.

- Always remember to "first, do no harm." Do not hypoperfuse already ischemic organs; avoid rapid swings of blood pressure beyond the already dysfunctional range of autoregulation of tissue perfusion. Consider contraindications to and side effects of specific medications. Coordinate the choice of pharmacotherapy among the many medical specialists involved in the care of the patient because each must share in the therapeutic goals and be familiar with the treatments used.

This article does not provide specific medication dosing guidelines. Rather, Table 3 summarizes therapeutic goals, suggested classes of agents used in various clinical scenarios, risks, caveats, and clinical "pearls" as they apply to the common clinical presentations of hypertensive emergency.

Hypertensive urgency and severe hypertension

Significant hypertension, typically SBP > 180 mm Hg or DBP > 110 mm Hg corresponding to stage III hypertension in JNC VI [1], without acutely evolving end-organ damage is a much more common presentation than a hypertensive emergency. This condition is described traditionally as a hypertensive urgency; however, this terminology represents a psychologic "framing effect" [12] that presumes this condition needs to be treated urgently. In fact, there is a substantial body of evidence that the rapid control of asymptomatic hypertension often results in adverse effects. Faced with a patient whose initial history and physical examination do not suggest emergent end-organ damage, consider the following points before initiating therapy.

First, assess the accuracy of the blood pressure reading. To meet JNC VII [2] criteria for accuracy, two readings must be taken at least 5 minutes apart with the patient at rest in a seated position. Keep in mind that with any measurement there is a statistical tendency for repeat measurements to regress toward the mean. This mathematical principle has been validated in a study of 195 consecutive hypertensive patients in an emergency department that documented a mean decline of 11.6 mm Hg in repeated diastolic blood pressure readings [13]. Remember also to repeat unexpectedly high blood pressure readings as a measurement error that can arise from the misapplication of the sphygmomanometer cuff, use of an undersized cuff, or operator error [14]. Even in the most technologically sophisticated settings, there is still a need for a manual sphygmomanometer with a variety of cuff sizes.

Second, consider whether the hypertension is reactive. If the hypertension is caused by anxiety, pain, use of sympathomimetics as innocent as decongestants or as risky as cocaine, or by withdrawal states such as alcohol or discontinuation of antihypertensive medication, addressing the underlying condition is the first priority.

Third, determine whether the elevation represents ongoing severe hypertension or a temporary perturbation. A study of patients who were hypertensive during an emergency department visit showed that, at follow-up clinic visits, only 69% of those with initial readings of 140 to 159 mm Hg SBP or 90 to

Table 3
Common presenting scenarios of hypertensive emergency

Modes of comparison	Hypertensive encephalopathy, cerebrovascular accident, intracranial hemorrhage	Acute congestive heart failure or pulmonary edema	Acute myocardial infarction or acute coronary syndrome	Aortic dissection	Acute cocaine or sympathomimetic intoxication
Therapeutic goal	• First do no harm, avoid hypoperfusion • Do not exceed 20% reduction of BP	• Reduction of BP, especially by vasodilatation • Promote diuresis	• Reduction of BP • Decrease myocardial oxygen demand	• Reduction of shear forces by reduction of BP and tachycardia	• Reduction of excessive sympathomemetic drive
Suggested agents	• Nicardipine: reduces cerebral ischemia • Consider ultra short acting agents (esmolol or nitroprusside)	• IV nitroglycerin • Morphine • IV angiotensin converting enzyme inhibitor • IV diuretic	• IV β blocker • IV nitroglycerin	• IV labetalol • IV β blocker • Nitroprusside	• Benzodiazepine • IV nitroglycerin • IV labetalol
Risk of therapy	• Cerebral autoregulation is disrupted in the ischemic brain • Patients demonstrate marked lability of BP with any agent, and hypoperfusion of the brain can occur	• Diuretics and angiotensin converting enzyme inhibitor can exacerbate renal dysfunction	• β Blockade can exacerbate left ventricular failure	• Nitroprusside is extremely potent and requires continuous intra-arterial BP monitoring	• Unopposed β blockade can cause alpha storm and increase cocaine toxicity
Pearls	• There is no clear evidence of benefit with intensive control of BP in the setting of stroke	• Diuretics are slow to work • Angiotensin converting enzyme inhibitor has rapid onset of action • IV nitrates dilate capacitance vessels at low doses, higher doses dilate arterioles and lower BP	• β Blockade also reduces mortality associated with ventricular arrhythmia	• Avoid volume depletion in patients requiring IV dye or going for general anesthesia	• Measure core temperature and treat hyperthermia if present • Consider the possibility of multidrug use

99 mm Hg DBP remained hypertensive but 100% correlation of subsequent readings in patients who had > 180 mm Hg SBP or > 110 mm Hg DBP [15].

If all of the above criteria are met, the presence of severe hypertension is confirmed, but the issue of urgency remains. At this juncture, many patients are referred for urgent evaluation, including EKG, urinalysis, blood glucose and hematocrit, serum potassium, creatinine (or estimated glomerular filtration rate), and calcium, as recommended in the JNC VII report [2]. The results of this testing are used to identify compelling indications for the use of individual drug classes. That this testing is appropriate is indisputable; that it identifies urgency is doubtful. Many patients who have significant hypertension will have chronic EKG abnormalities such as left ventricular hypertrophy, a strain pattern or T-wave inversion, but in the absence of symptoms, these findings seldom warrant acute intervention. Likewise, many of these patients will have a degree of renal impairment, usually found to be chronic and without the need for immediate intervention. These patients should be treated, according to JNC guidelines for stage II hypertension, with two oral agents, as described in Table 4.

Thus far in this discussion of severe hypertension, the issue of urgency remains unresolved. Are there symptoms or situations that differentiate urgency from severe asymptomatic hypertension? In terms of symptoms, concern arises over patients who present with nonspecific headache, without other signs of central nervous system emergency. There are no studies that document headache alone, which can be mitigated by immediate treatment, as a risk factor for further complication. Although many clinicians take advantage of the patient's perception of the need to treat headache in the setting of severe hypertension, it is preferable to initiate treatment with a regimen consistent with long-term use. In a large study [16] of nonemergent severe hypertension in an emergency department setting, 269 of 11,531 (2.3%) of patients had systolic blood pressure > 180 mm Hg or diastolic blood pressure > 110 mm Hg. The most frequent chief complaints were musculoskeletal pain in 18% and headache in 12%. Only 56 of the 269 were treated acutely, usually with a calcium channel-blocking drug.

Table 4
Compelling indications for individual drug classes

Compelling indication	Initial therapy options
Heart failure	THIAZ, BB, ACEI, ARB, ALDO ANT
Post-myocardial infarction	BB, ACEI, ALDO ANT
High CVD risk	THIAZ, BB, ACEI, CCB
Diabetes	THIAZ, BB, ACEI, ARB, CCB
Chronic kidney disease	ACEI, ARB
Recurrent stroke prevention	THIAZ, ACEI

Abbreviations: ACEI, angiotensin converting enzyme inhibitor; ALDO ANT, aldosterone antagonist; ARB, angiotensin receptor blocker; BB, β blocker; CCB, calcium channel blocker; THIAZ, thiazide.

The strongest correlation to decision to treat was not the symptoms but the severity of blood pressure reading. In most cases, the patient's home regimen was not altered. This typical pattern of care argues that most clinicians do not place special priority on the treatment of nonspecific headache.

In terms of situations that denote urgency, an argument for immediate treatment can be mounted if patients need urgent procedural evaluation or intervention. Patients who have uncontrolled hypertension are known to have labile blood pressures under general anesthesia, and IV pharmacotherapy will often be needed during anesthesia [17]; therefore, it makes sense to initiate control preprocedure. Preoperative β blockade has demonstrated benefit in lowering perioperative complications, especially in hypertensive patients who have other risk factors for cardiovascular disease [18]. In contrast to the absence of a proven benefit of emergent treatment of severe asymptomatic hypertension, there is substantial evidence of morbidity resulting from rapidly lowering blood pressure in the chronically hypertensive patient. Of particular concern are reports that demonstrate the occurrence of stroke with both aggressive [19,20] and moderately acute blood pressure reduction [20]. In addition, symptomatic hypotension, myocardial infarction, and even death have occurred from oral agents used to acutely lower blood pressure [21–23].

Because of the lack of proven benefit and substantial evidence of risk in rapid blood pressure lowering, the present authors suggest that most cases of severe hypertension should be treated according to JNC VII [2] guidelines for the selection of medication that produces timely but gradual improvement in blood pressure control. Instead of initiating rapid control of blood pressure, emergency care should emphasize the thoughtful initiation of long-term therapy and appropriate follow-up care. The widely accepted guidelines for acceptable timeline in hypertensive management have been adapted from JNC VI (Table 5) [1].

In an editorial, Matthews [24] addresses the urge to treat the asymptomatic hypertensive aggressively: "The principle 'FIRST, DO NO HARM' is applicable. The compulsive need to treat reaches the pathological in some physicians, especially during the early years in their careers. If the urge to treat asymptomatic hypertension becomes over whelming, use an agent

Table 5
Appropriate follow up and intervention for asymptomatic patients without major end-organ damage

BP (mm Hg)	Follow up
140–159/90–99	Observe and confirm within 2 mo
160–179/100–109	Confirm and treat within 1 mo
180–209/110–119	Confirm and treat within 1 wk
210+/120+	Confirm, evaluate, and initiate therapy immediately with close follow up

Data from National Heart, Lung, and Blood Institute. Seventh report of the Joint National Committee on Prevention, Detection, Evaluation, and Treatment of High Blood Pressure. Publication no. NIH 03-5233. Bethesda (MD): NIH; 2003.

that lowers blood pressure gradually over time and ensure the patient understands the need and has an opportunity for early and adequate follow-up. This approach should be safe for the patient and will satisfy the concern that you will be sued if you do nothing. For the majority of these patients, ensuring good follow-up as an outpatient will suffice."

Summary

Remember to treat patients, not numbers. Use fast acting short-term medicines only when convincing evidence of rapidly evolving end-organ damage is present. For all patients, emergent or asymptomatic, the treatment goal is long-term control of hypertension. Potent IV agents for the immediate control of elevated blood pressure need to be used cautiously, bearing in mind both the side effects and the hazards of overly rapid control of hypertension. Conventional oral medication regimens demonstrated to modify the risks of chronic hypertension should be used whenever possible and as early as is practical to promote gradual control of hypertension. Whenever a patient presents for the evaluation of severe hypertension in an emergent setting, take the opportunity to encourage appropriate ongoing follow-up; after all, hypertension is not a single episode, it is an ongoing threat to good health.

References

[1] National Heart, Lung, and Blood Institute. Sixth report of the Joint National Committee on Prevention, Detection, Evaluation, and Treatment of High Blood Pressure (JNC VI). Available at: http://www.nhlbi.nih.gov/guidelines/hypertension/jnc6.PDF. Accessed January 8, 2006.
[2] National Heart, Lung, and Blood Institute. Seventh report of the Joint National Committee on Prevention, Detection, Evaluation, and Treatment of High Blood Pressure (JNC VII); 2003. Publication no. NIH 03–5233. Bethesda (MD): NIH; 2003.
[3] Keith NM, Wagner HP, Barker NW. Some different types of essential hypertension and their course and prognosis. Am J Med Sci 1939;197:332–43.
[4] Fuchs FP, Maestri MK, Bredemeior M, et al. Study of usefulness of optic fundi examination of patients with hypertension in a clinical setting. J Hum Hypertens 1995;9:547–51.
[5] Webster J, Petrie JC, Jeffers TA, et al. Accelerated hypertension-patterns of mortality and clinical factors affecting outcome in treated patients. Q J Med 1993;86:485–93.
[6] Calhoun DA, Oparil S. Treatment of hypertensive crisis. N Engl J Med 1990;323:1177–83.
[7] Ault MJ, Ellrodt AG. Pathophysiologic events leading to the end organ effects of acute hypertension. Am J Emerg Med 1985;3:10–5.
[8] Strandgaard S, Paulson OB. Cerebral autoregulation. Stroke 1984;709:413–6.
[9] Zampaglione B, Pascale C, Marchisio M, et al. Hypertensive urgencies and emergencies: prevalence and clinical presentation. Hypertension 1996;27:144–7.
[10] Messerli FH. This day 50 years ago. N Engl J Med 1995;332:1038–9.
[11] Calhoun DA, Oparil S. Hypertensive crisis since FDR: a partial victory. N Engl J Med 1995; 332:1029–30.
[12] Redelmeier DA. Improving patient care.The cognitive psychology of missed diagnoses. Ann Intern Med 2005;142(2):115–20.

[13] Pitts SR, Adams RP. Emergency department hypertension and regression to the mean. Ann Emerg Med 1998;31:214–8.

[14] Hla KM, Vokaty KA, Feussner JR. Overestimation of diastolic blood pressure in the elderly: magnitude of the problem and a potential solution. J Am Geriatr Soc 1985;33:659–63.

[15] Daniel N. the validity of emergency department triage blood pressure measurements. Acad Emerg Med 2004;11:237–43.

[16] Chiang WK, Jamshahi B. Asymptomatic hypertension in the ED. Am J Emerg Med 1998;16: 701–4.

[17] Eagle KA, Berger PB, Calkins SH, et al. ACC/AHA guideline update for perioperative cardiovascular evaluation for noncardiac surgery: executive summary. Circulation 2002;105: 1257–67.

[18] Mangano DT, Layug EL, Wallace A, et al. Effects of atenolol on mortality and cardiovascular morbidity after noncardiac surgery. N Engl J Med 1996;335:1713–20.

[19] Grossman E, Masserli FH, Grodzicki T, et al. Should a moratorium be placed on sublingual nifedipine capsules given for hypertensive emergencies and pseudoemergencies? JAMA 1996;276:3128–31.

[20] Yanturali S, Akay S, Ayrik C, et al. Adverse events associated with aggressive treatment of increased blood pressure. Int J Clin Pract 2004;58:517–9.

[21] Fischberg GM, Lozano E. Rajamanik, et al. Stroke precipitated by moderate blood pressure reduction. J Emerg Med 2000;19:339–46.

[22] Oei SG, Oei SK, Brolmann HA. Myocardial infarction during nifedipine therapy for preterm labor. N Engl J Med 1999;100:959–61.

[23] Sheir JG, Howland MA, Hoffman RS. Fatality from administration of labelalol and crushed extended release nifedipine. Ann Pharmacother 2003;37:1420–3.

[24] Matthews J. The hypertensive patient in the emergency department. J Emerg Med 2000; 19:379.

ELSEVIER
SAUNDERS

Med Clin N Am 90 (2006) 453–479

THE MEDICAL
CLINICS
OF NORTH AMERICA

Dyspnea

Joseph R. Shiber, MD[a,b,c,*], Jose Santana, MD[b]

[a]Department of Medicine, East Carolina University, Greenville, NC, USA
[b]Department of Emergency Medicine, East Carolina University, Greenville, NC, USA
[c]Emergency Medicine–Internal Medicine Combined Residency, East Carolina University,
Greenville, NC, USA

The sensation of breathlessness, dyspnea, is clinically important when it is recognized by the patient as abnormal. The development of shortness of breath (SOB) or the inability to satisfy oxygen requirements is an expected outcome of overexertion, such as occurs after running or heavy lifting. When dyspnea occurs at rest or during exertion that is less than expected, it is considered pathologic and a symptom of a disease state. Multiple organ systems are involved in the differential diagnosis of dyspnea, most commonly the cardiovascular and pulmonary systems. The type and severity of underlying lung or heart disease have been shown to correlate with the description offered by the patient [1,2]. Box 1 illustrates the extensive differential diagnosis for dyspnea.

The outpatient management of dyspnea has changed recently, with the advent of new diagnostic tests and therapies. These innovations have allowed the outpatient clinician to more accurately diagnose the underlying disorder and initiate appropriate therapy. Now, clinical decisions based on whether to continue outpatient management or admit a patient to the hospital can be augmented by treatment algorithms. This article constructs a decision and management protocol for physicians, allowing for a decision to treat the adult dyspneic patient in the office or transfer the patient to a hospital in pursuit of a confirmed diagnosis and definitive care. The first step is to begin with a rapid initial assessment of the airway, breathing, and circulation, while gathering a focused history and physical examination [3]. Once the initial examination and vital signs have been obtained and an emergent situation has been excluded, the patient can be placed in one of three categories: (1) distress with unstable vital signs; (2) distress with stable

* Corresponding author. Department of Medicine, East Carolina University, 600 Moye Boulevard, Greenville, NC 27834.
  E-mail address: shiberj@mail.ecu.edu (J.R. Shiber).

0025-7125/06/$ - see front matter © 2006 Elsevier Inc. All rights reserved.
doi:10.1016/j.mcna.2005.11.006
medical.theclinics.com

Box 1. Differential diagnosis for dyspnea

Mechanical interference with ventilation
Abdominal or chest mass
Asthma, emphysema, bronchitis
Endobronchial tumor
Interstitial fibrosis of any cause
Kyphoscoliosis
Left ventricular failure
Lymphangitic tumor
Obesity
Obstruction to airflow, central or peripheral
Pleural thickening
Resistance to expansion of the chest wall or diaphragm
Resistance to expansion of the lung
Thoracic burn with eschar formation
Tracheal or laryngeal stenosis

Weakness of the respiratory pump
Absolute
Hyperinflation
Neuromuscular disease
Obesity
Pleural effusion
Pneumothorax
Previous poliomyelitis
Relative

Increased respiratory drive
Decreased cardiac output
Decreased effective hemoglobin
Hypoxemia of any cause
Metabolic acidosis
Renal disease
Stimulation of intrapulmonary receptors

Wasted ventilation
Capillary destruction
Large-vessel obstruction

Psychologic dysfunction
Anxiety
Bodily preoccupation, somatization disorder
Depression
Secondary gain, malingering

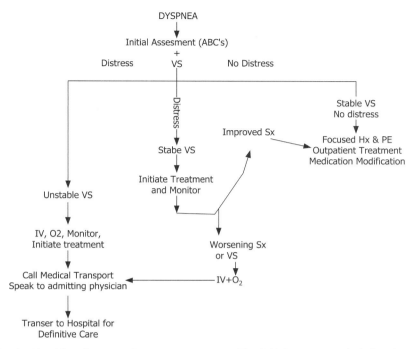

Fig. 1. Algorithm for acute dyspnea management. The initial assessment includes airway, breathing, and circulation (ABC's), a brief history of the present illness, medical history, medications, and allergies. Hx, history; Sx, symptoms; VS, vital signs.

vital signs; or (3) no distress and stable vital signs. Following this algorithm, a patient's disposition can be determined expeditiously (Fig. 1).

Acute myocardial infarction (AMI) and congestive heart failure (CHF) are the most common cardiovascular disorders that lead to dyspnea. Patients who have had an AMI usually describe retrosternal chest discomfort and an inability to catch their breath. This sensation occurs secondary to a reduction in cardiac output and pulmonary perfusion and is caused by reduced contractility of the ischemic or stunned myocardium. The administration of supplemental oxygen, therapy to decrease myocardial oxygen consumption and increase coronary vasodilation, and the use of revascularization strategies such as fibrinolytic therapy or percutaneous coronary intervention may readily relieve the symptoms. Patients who have an exacerbation of congestive heart failure may describe a sensation of SOB with exertion, orthopnea, and paroxysmal nocturnal dyspnea. Symptoms generally resolve or are improved by giving the patient supplemental oxygen, diuretics, therapy aimed at decreasing preload and afterload, and medical or surgical treatments to improve cardiac contractility. Pulmonary dyspnea is commonly caused by chronic obstructive pulmonary disease (COPD), asthma, pneumothorax, and pneumonia. Chronic obstructive pulmonary disease and asthma are considered obstructive processes that may produce chronic SOB punctuated by sudden acute worsening of symptoms. Often, the treatment of these diseases requires the use of steroids and inhaled bronchodilators to resolve the ensuing exacerbation. Table 1 describes the symptoms of dyspnea according to the disease state. Primary care clinicians should always consider other life-threatening causes of SOB such as pulmonary embolism (PE).

Although many of the causes that lead to dyspnea will be treated ultimately in the causes or inpatient ward, primary care physicians should be knowledgeable about the subtle and atypical presentations of potentially life-threatening diagnoses.

Congestive heart failure

Congestive heart failure is one of the most common causes of dyspnea seen in health care settings. Approximately 1.2% to 2% of the population in the United States has heart failure, and most patients (75%–80%) are older than 65 years of age. It has been estimated that approximately 20 million people unknowingly have depressed left ventricular function in the absence of symptoms and are likely to become symptomatic within a 1- to 5-year period. Patients who have CHF visit physicians more than 11 million times per year and are responsible for 3.5 million hospitalizations per year, with one third requiring rehospitalization within 3 months after discharge [4].

Patients may present to an outpatient clinic as an established, well-known patient with CHF or as a first-time visitor. Thus, primary care physicians are on the front line when it comes to tentatively diagnosing congestive heart failure. The well-established patient usually has been diagnosed previously with heart failure or has significant predisposing risk factors, such as hypertension or coronary artery disease (CAD). The patient who is newly diagnosed with CHF presents the added challenge of tailoring the outpatient workup and investigation for the cause of the disease. The diagnosis is determined after a full history, physical examination, and diagnostic studies have been performed. Once the diagnosis and severity of illness are determined, the appropriate treatment can be initiated. In many cases, patients who present to an outpatient clinic will be too ill to be taken care of in the office and will require transfer to an emergency department (ED) for a definitive diagnosis, treatment, and possibly admission to the hospital.

Table 1
Symptoms associated with diagnosis

Diagnosis	Symptoms
CHF	Dyspnea on exertion, paroxymal nocturnal dypnea, orthopnea
AMI	Radiating chest pressure, diaphoresis, SOB
PE	Fever, pleuritic chest pain, sudden onset SOB, syncope
COPD/asthma	Cough, smoker, SOB relieved with nebulizer or MDI
Pneumonia	Fever, productive cough, SOB
Pneumothorax	Sudden onset pleuritic chest pain, SOB not relieved with O_2

History

The patient's history will help determine what elements of the physical examination will aid in the appropriate diagnosis and what diagnostic studies may or may not be indicated. The onset, severity, duration, alleviating, aggravating, and associated symptoms are all pertinent to the history. To illustrate, consider the following case: A 55-year-old man presents to his primary care physicians clinic with a medical history significant for hypertension, with the chief complaint, "I'm unable to walk very far without becoming winded." He states that he now uses three pillows to keep from feeling short of breath and wakes up frequently at night to catch his breath, and he has noticed that his legs are swollen.

This patient is like many of the people seen everyday in outpatient clinics. How is the practitioner to sort out this patient from the other patients seen the same day with similar complaints? Simply, it is all in the history. The important information to obtain includes onset, duration of symptoms, what activities result in SOB, and any other associated symptoms. In addition, the history should focus on the other deadly causes of SOB. Has the patient just taken a 10-hour plane ride? Has there been any associated chest pain, back pain, nausea, or diaphoresis? Has the patient experienced palpitations or any other symptoms?

It is also important to ask the patient about their medical, surgical, social, and family history to determine risk factors and possible causes, and ask about medication use and record the current dosage to initiate or modify treatments.

Physical examination

The physical examination should be given due importance, despite innovations in objective laboratory and radiographic tests. Studies have shown that the physical examination depends on the diagnosis and prognosis of congestive heart failure. The physical examination begins the first moment the patient is encountered, during which their general appearance is observed. A person's appearance speaks volumes about the severity of their dyspnea. A patient who becomes short of breath after a few steps in the office is obviously very different from the one who can walk half of a mile before becoming dyspneic. This categorization can be further described by using the New Heart Association's Functional Classification of Heart Failure. Rating the patient on this functional scale from I to V can be used as a comparison to the previous functional status, determine the acuity of change in an established patient, and the response to treatment [5]. The patient's disposition can often be determined by the initial general appearance; whether the patient can be treated with oral medication or he or she requires transportation to the ED for intravenous (IV) medication administration and hospital admission.

It is imperative to record and review the patient's initial vital signs, including pulse oximetry, and to repeat assessments after interventions.

Obtaining an accurate body weight to compare with previous values, particularly if the patient weighs him/herself regularly, will suggest whether there has been a recent increase in weight. Tachypnea, tachycardia, and hypoxia are expected findings during a CHF exacerbation. Hypertension may be secondary to stress or present as a cause of failure; if hypotension is present, cardiac output is likely to be severely decreased. If hypotension and tachycardia are present, the physician must consider cardiogenic shock with inadequate tissue perfusion. Ideally, this type of patient will be recognized immediately, and stabilization can begin as urgent supervised transportation to the hospital emergency department is arranged.

After the initial observation, the clinician should work through a systematic evaluation. An examination of the neck may show jugular venous distention, indicating increased intravascular volume or right-sided filling pressures. Palpation and auscultation of the carotids may demonstrate signs of atherosclerotic disease, which may indicate that other vascular beds, such as the coronary vessels, are involved with disease. An examination of the lungs may reveal the presence of rales or crackles from pulmonary edema and wheezing from bronchial and interstitial edema. Decreased tactile fremitus on palpation and dullness on percussion indicate pleural effusion. An S_3 gallop found on cardiac auscultation represents left ventricular systolic dysfunction, whereas an S_4 is associated with left ventricular diastolic dysfunction with acute cardiac ischemia being the most worrisome cause. An irregular heart rhythm may be detected that may indicate that an underlying arrhythmia is present, or a new murmur may signal acute valvular dysfunction. Quiet heart sounds may also be detected in some cases and be caused by a pericardial effusion.

An abdominal examination may demonstrate findings secondary to congestion of the hepatic venous system, resulting in hepatomegaly and jugular distension (hepatojugular reflex) when depressing the liver edge. Ascites can also be observed by a fluid wave on palpation. The extremities should be evaluated for perfusion, including an assessment of skin color and temperature, peripheral pulses, and capillary refill. Lower extremity pitting edema is a sign of right-sided heart failure, whereas decreased hair growth on the lower extremity is indicative of chronic edema (Table 2).

Diagnostic studies

Heart failure can be diagnosed by the history and constellation of clinical findings alone, but imaging and laboratory studies may be necessary to help confirm the definitive diagnosis as well as to stratify the severity of the episode. The availability of these tests varies from the primary care office to the urgent care setting. Pulse oximetry should be the first diagnostic modality used while taking the vital signs. Based on these data, the patient's level of oxygenation and the reversibility of the disease process can be determined. If a heart failure patient presents with symptomatic hypoxia that is not improved with supplemental oxygen, this patient falls under the

Table 2
Physical examination of dyspnea

Diagnosis	Findings
CHF	Edema, jugular venous distension, S3 or S4, hepatojugular reflux, murmurs, rales, wheezing, hypertension
ACS	Tachycardia, heart failure findings
PE	Wheezing, lower extremity swelling, friction rub
COPD/asthma	Wheezing, barrel chest, clubbing, decreased breath sounds, pulsus paradoxical, accessory muscle use
Pneumonia	Fever, crackles, increased fremitus
Pneumothorax	Absent breath sounds, hyperesonance, jugular venous distension, tracheal deviation

category of unstable and is in distress. In this category, the immediate transfer to the hospital is required. Patients who have chronic hypoxia are eligible for home oxygen therapy if their oxygenation on exertion falls below 88%, with coverage by private insurance and government agencies [6].

ECG is an invaluable tool and should be performed early on all patients being evaluated for SOB. The ECG may help determine the cause of heart failure and help define the anatomic location of CAD. Ischemic heart disease may be interpreted on the ECG as an ST-segment depression or a T-wave inversion, whereas an ST-segment elevation or Q waves indicate previous infarction. Patients may also have arrhythmias and signs of electrolyte deficiency or excess. In the case of hypokalemia and hyperkalemia, flattened T waves or U waves, or both, and peaked T waves may be found, respectively. Ventricular and atrial enlargement can be determined as anatomical features of heart failure by using recognized ECG criteria. Low QRS voltages, noted in precordial leads, are caused commonly by pericardial effusion, infiltrative heart disease, COPD, hypothyroidism, and obesity. Chest radiographs (CXR) are used to look for pulmonary vascular congestion, interstitial fluid, and pulmonary edema. The presence of cardiomegaly indicates that the process did not occur suddenly, but differentiating the pericardial silhouette from the cardiac contour can be challenging by chest radiography. Echocardiography is the most important noninvasive modality with which to determine systolic and diastolic function, ventricular size, the presence of valvular disease, and the presence of pericardial effusion. Systolic heart failure is identified by a decreased ejection fraction and dilated chambers, whereas diastolic heart failure is more difficult to diagnose and less common than systolic dysfunction. These patients have a normal or elevated ejection fraction but reduced diastolic filling caused by impaired myocardial relaxation, and they have a specific secondary cause, such as hypertension or aortic stenosis.

Laboratory studies can add to the objective findings. Anemia can be found in chronic heart failure, and polycythemia may be encountered in those with chronic hypoxic states. A high platelet count can be an acute phase reactant, whereas for older fragile heart failure patients, pneumonia may cause an exacerbation and present with a high white blood cell count. The measurement of serum digoxin level is important in patients taking this drug because of the relatively narrow therapeutic index. Prerenal acute renal failure can be determined by finding an elevated blood urea nitrogen (BUN) level, and increased BUN-creatinine ratio, indicating hypoperfusion of the kidneys. Obtaining serum values of potassium, magnesium, calcium, sodium, chloride, and bicarbonate may assist in determining intravascular volume status, whereas replacing depleted electrolytes may reduce the risk of cardiac arrhythmia. Brain natriuretic peptide (BNP) is a cardiac neuro-hormone secreted by the cardiac ventricles in response to ventricular wall tension, pressure overload, and increased volume expansion. BNP can now be detected rapidly by a simple laboratory test, which is becoming more readily available in the outpatient setting. This value allows for a more definitive diagnosis of heart failure by narrowing the differential for dyspnea. If this value is elevated by ≥ 100 pg/mL, the high sensitivity and specificity of this test allows for accurate diagnosis of heart failure. Values that are ≤ 100 pg/mL reliably rule out depressed left ventricular function [7,8]. Brain natriuretic peptide has also been used as a predictor of mortality and can be used to follow improvement after CHF therapy in cases of acute cardiac decompensation and for outpatients. The assessment of BNP values over time allows the clinician to better estimate an exacerbation based on an individualized value. BNP produces vasodilation, diuresis, and natriuresis, and inhibits the renin-angiotensin-aldosterone axis. Although BNP is an available medication, nesiritide (recombinant human BNP), its IV formulation, has been limited to inpatient use for severely decompensated CHF.

Management

The initial management of CHF begins after the patient has been evaluated quickly and the level of acuteness has been determined. Using the categories described earlier, patients are treated according to their specific category. If the patient is in acute distress, they should receive supplemental oxygen and preload reduction with sublingual, transcutaneous, or IV nitroglycerin (NTG). Have them remain with their head elevated but their feet dependent, as in a reverse-Trendelenburg position, to further discourage venous return. Oral or IV furosemide is recommended if the patient has evidence of volume overload. If the blood pressure is still elevated, the reduction in cardiac afterload should be accomplished with an arterial vasodilator, such as an angiotensin-converting enzyme inhibitor or hydralazine. The use of calcium channel blockers should be avoided in patients who have CHF caused by reduced systolic function, and β-blockers should not be used while the patient is in a decompensated episode. Obviously, many of these patients will require transportation to the nearest ED for definitive care.

These patients are further classified into unstable and stable based on vital signs. Unstable patient are initially given therapy while arrangements are made for transfer to an inpatient facility. Stable patients, after initial treatment, can be observed for improvement; but if they become unstable, follow the same algorithm as above. The patients who improve significantly can be managed much in the same way as those that are initially found to be in no acute distress. These patients benefit from home instruction and education, medication modification, and close follow-up (Table 3).

Table 3
Distress classification and management

Disease	No acute distress	Acute distress	Initial treatment	
			Stable	Unstable
CHF	No dyspnea at rest	Dyspnea at rest or minimal exertion	Furosemide po, Bp control, O_2	Furosemide IV, NTG, Bp control, O_2
CAD	Stable angina	Acute chest pain, diaphoresis, tachycardia or bradycardia, hypotension or hypertension, syncope	ASA, NTG, O_2, analgesia	ASA, NTG, O_2, analgesia, $\pm$ plavix
PE	Asymptomatic silent	Dyspnea at rest, fever, hypoxia, tachycardia, hypertension	NA	LMWH, O_2, analgesics
Pneumonia	Normal O_2 saturation, mild dyspnea, low PORT score	Decreased O_2 saturation, functional debilitating dyspnea, tachycardia, high/moderate PORT score	O_2, acetominophen, antibiotics po	O_2, acetominophen, IM or IV antibiotics
Pneumothorax	Spontaneous	Tension	Analgesics	Needle decompression, O_2, analgesics
COPD/asthma	>80% peak flow	<80% peak flow	O_2, MDI treatment	O_2, MDI, or nebulizer treatment and steroids

Abbreviations: ASA, aspirin; Bp, blood pressure; IM, intramuscular; LMWH, low molecular weight heparin; NA, not applicable; po, by mouth.
Data from Steering Committee and Membership of the Advisory Council to Improve Outcomes Nationwide in Heart Failure. Am J Cardiol 1999;83(Suppl 2A);1A–39A.

Acute coronary syndrome

CAD is the leading cause of death in the United States, caused acutely by myocardial infarction and as a result of chronic problems such as congestive heart failure. It is estimated that 13.7 million people in the United States suffer from CAD, with half having myocardial infarction and the other half suffering from chronic angina [9]. An acute coronary syndrome (ACS) refers to the rupture of an atherosclerotic plaque with the activation of platelets and fibrin, resulting in thrombus formation and either reduced flow or the occlusion of a coronary artery. Many of these individuals have significant risk factors identified before an acute event by their primary medical providers; thus it is important for a physician in an outpatient environment to recognize patients who have acute dyspnea caused by acute coronary syndrome, so that prompt initial treatment can be started and transport initiated as soon as possible. The goal is for no more than 30 minutes to elapse from the time of initial contact until emergency medical services are called or appropriate measures are instituted [10]. Once the patient arrives at the hospital, the goal is 90 minutes from door to reperfusion, in an attempt to limit the myocardial ischemia and injury to 2 hours or less [11]. Another consideration is that some patients, particularly women and the elderly, may present with atypical presentations of AMI, particularly isolated dyspnea. If an acute coronary syndrome is suspected, transport for definitive management should not be delayed.

History

The rapid assessment of dyspnea in acute coronary syndrome is initiated with a brief targeted interview and risk-factor stratification. If the patient has had a syncopal event or has unstable vital signs, the initial assessment starts with an evaluation of airway, breathing, and circulation, while taking a brief history. It is necessary to distinguish an ACS patient from a patient who simply has stable chronic angina, which does not have the same underlying pathophysiology or associated morbidity or mortality and therefore does not require the same aggressive therapies.

Patients who complain of acute dyspnea and have acute coronary syndrome often describe left-sided retrosternal chest pressure, diaphoresis, tachycardia, radiation of pain to the jaw, neck, or left or right arm, and nausea. These symptoms may last several minutes and be alleviated by sublingual NTG and aggravated by exertion. Importantly, a large percentage of cardiac ischemic episodes may not have these specific symptoms [11]. It has also been documented that up to one third of myocardial infarction patients have no chest pain on presentation to the hospital [12]. These patients may not be diagnosed initially or at all, allowing for myocardial damage to exceed that of an otherwise treated patient. Therefore, a thorough history that includes past medical, surgical, social, and family history must be obtained so that those individuals with vague symptoms or several risk factors can be evaluated appropriately.

Risk factors for CAD include male age ≥ 45 years, female age ≥ 55 years, diabetes, obesity, a family history for CAD, tobacco use, hypertension, a history of atherosclerotic disease, hypertriglyceridemia, high levels of low-density lipoprotein cholesterol, and low levels of high-density lipoprotein (HDL) cholesterol (≤ 40 mg/dL). High HDL (≥ 60 mg/dL) is a negative risk factor, which should be considered [13].

Physical examination

The physical examination should focus on the cardiovascular and respiratory systems. The examination will follow the same general sequence as for congestive heart failure. Specific attention should be devoted to cardiac auscultation. An S_4 sound may indicate ventricular stiffness caused by ischemic stunning, and a new murmur may represent acute valvular dysfunction, causing regurgitation or, less commonly, rupture of the interventricular septum, allowing for a new left-to-right shunt. Quiet heart sounds and other evidence of a symptomatic pericardial effusion may be caused by ventricular free wall rupture, causing acute hemopericardium. Those patients presenting with unstable vital signs in acute distress will first require rapid evaluation of airway, breathing, and circulation.

Diagnosis

The diagnosis of acute myocardial infarction is based on signs and symptoms, diagnostic electrocardiographic criteria, and an elevation of cardiac biomarkers. Because the latter usually can be performed only in the hospital, outpatient criteria are limited to ECG changes and patient presentation. Other diagnostic tools in an inpatient facility may include further blood work, echocardiography, and chest radiography. Relief of chest pain quickly after receiving supplemental oxygen, soluble aspirin, or sublingual NTG, is suggestive but not specific for acute CAD, but it should not be used as diagnostic criteria to confirm or exclude an ACS.

Laboratory tests may demonstrate anemia as the cause of the ischemia or infarction. As described above, electrolytes may be deficient or in excess and predispose to cardiac arrhythmias, which decrease blood flow while increasing demands on the myocardium. Rapid assays of the cardiac isomer of creatine phosphokinase and troponin are becoming more available, and although the assays are very sensitive and specific for cardiac injury, serum levels require a minimum of several hours to rise during an acute coronary event. The ECG may demonstrate many types of changes that indicate ischemia or injury and infarction. Typical changes include hyperacute T waves, T-wave inversion, ST-segment elevation, Q waves, or new onset left bundle branch blocks in infarction and ST-segment depression in ischemia. It is important to identify the region of the myocardium that is affected when evaluating an ECG. An echocardiogram can be used to identify wall motion abnormalities. This information, along with the anatomical description of myocardial damage by ECG, will provide important information to the cardiac interventionalist when deciding which coronary artery to image first on percutaneous coronary catheterization.

Management

When patients who have acute dyspnea present and ACS is suspected or diagnosed, prompt initial therapy and transfer for further evaluation and definitive treatment are required. An IV line should be started, and the patient should be placed on a cardiac monitor. Therapy begins with the administration of oxygen, rapidly absorbed soluble aspirin (not enteric coated), and sublingual NTG (0.4 mg). If the patient develops hypotension in response to NTG, an IV bolus of crystalloid should be given, and further NTG must be used cautiously [14,15]. A β-blocker should be given to patients without bradycardia or heart block to decrease myocardial oxygen consumption [16]. The transfer of a patient suspected of having ACS should not be impeded by further examinations, studies, or treatment. The goal is to obtain definitive treatment through reperfusion as soon as possible (see Table 3).

One of the most important skills in the outpatient setting is in recognizing and diagnosing an atypical acute coronary syndrome. Patients known to have subtle, atypical, and even silent myocardial infarctions include the elderly and diabetics. Female patients have also been found to present with atypical presentations. Primary care physicians should be on the alert for these types of presentations in their patients.

Pulmonary embolism

PE is one of the most commonly missed lethal diagnoses. Untreated PE has a mortality rate from 18% to 35% and therefore should always be considered in the differential diagnosis of acute dyspnea [17]. In the United States, 1 in 1000 Americans is affected each year, making this disease a common clinical entity that can be treated if identified correctly. Of the 600,000 episodes of PE that occur each year, 50 to 100,000 patients die as a result of the disease [18]. Once the disease is diagnosed and treated, the incidence of recurrence and death is significantly reduced. The strategy in an outpatient clinic should be to immediately send any patient with significant clinical suspicion to the hospital emergency department for a definitive diagnosis and possible treatment. Because the objective data may not be available in the outpatient clinic, clinical suspicion is highly regarded as sufficient evidence to disposition early for definitive management. Considering that most deaths are attributed to the failure to diagnose, a quick, definitive diagnosis and management are imperative.

History

The history in patients who have PE may be misleading because the signs and symptoms are neither sensitive nor specific. An estimated 50% of cases of PE remain undiagnosed, underscoring the atypical nature of the disease [19]. The frequency of the most common signs and symptoms of PE have been studied. Dyspnea is the most common symptom, whereas tachypnea, pleuritic chest pain, and rales are also common signs and symptoms, at 73%, 70%, 66%, and 51%, respectively [20]. Other frequent symptoms include cough, hemoptysis, syncope, and fever. Although these symptoms are common in PE, they lack diagnostic sensitivity and specificity. It has been shown that patients who do not have PE have a similar frequency of symptoms [21].

It is important to inquire about any recent unilateral leg swelling, warmth, redness, or pain because lower extremity deep venous thrombosis (DVT) is the most common cause of PE. Risk-factor stratification is an important tool in gathering evidence to support suspicion of PE. Factors identified include immobilization, surgery within the past 3 months, stroke, history of venous thromboembolism, and malignancy [20]. Less common risk factors include increasing age, lower extremity trauma, extended travel, oral contraceptive pills, hormone replacement therapy, pregnancy, recent delivery, recent joint replacement, lower extremity fractures, and pelvic fractures. Other studies have added obesity, hypertension, severe CHF, pulmonary hypertension, and cigarette smoking. The medical and family history should also account for genetic or acquired causes of thrombophilia, including antithrombin III deficiency, lupus anticoagulant, protein C and S deficiency, factor V Leiden, and mutation in prothrombin G20210A, as well as nephrotic syndrome and inflammatory bowel disease.

Physical examination

A rapid examination of a dyspneic patient who has possible pulmonary thromboembolism is essential for disposition. The physical examination is used to further support a suspicious history and provides rapid support for the need to transport the patient to the ED. Vital signs may demonstrate fever, tachypnea, tachycardia, hypoxia, and hypotension. Of these findings, hypoxia is the most specific, although this can be masked by hyperventilation from a tachypneic patient. After the vital signs have been evaluated, the patient's general appearance is noted, followed by a focused cardiovascular and pulmonary physical examination. Patients who appear to be in acute distress may have rapid shallow breathing at rest, diaphoresis, and tachycardia. Their airway, breathing, and circulation should be assessed quickly, before they are transported to a hospital.

A focused respiratory examination consists of auscultation of the lungs. Examination findings may include normal, decreased breath sounds, a pleural friction rub, or rales. In patients who have pulmonary consolidation caused by an associated lung infarction, the presence of egophony can be appreciated on auscultation. Dullness to percussion and decreased tactile fremitus on palpation indicate a pleural effusion. Patients may also have reproducible chest pain on deep breathing. The cardiovascular examination may reveal signs of right-sided heart failure from pulmonary hypertension. Tachycardia, a right-sided S_4, and an increased pulmonic component of second heart sound may be auscultated. The remainder of the vascular examination consists of examining the lower extremities for signs of deep vein thrombosis as a possible cause. These examination findings include unilateral lower extremity edema, warmth, erythema, a palpable cord, and posterior leg pain on dorsiflexion of the ipsilateral foot.

Diagnosis

The diagnosis of PE is challenging because of vague, nonspecific symptoms or lack of symptoms. PE is diagnosed definitively by imaging studies, once the patient has been sent to the ED for evaluation. Laboratory tests, echocardiograms, and chest radiographs are modalities used to help provide supporting evidence but do not provide concrete evidence of PE. The diagnosis of a deep venous thromboembolism by ultrasonography may allow a clinician to assume PE is present with suggestive pulmonary symptoms or signs. Thus, a patient who is being evaluated for SOB who is found to have a DVT needs no further workup. The diagnosis is PE.

Laboratory test findings may be abnormal but are nonspecific. Leukocytosis can occur as a reactive phenomenon, as well as an elevated sedimentation rate. Respiratory alkalosis with an elevated A-a gradient is often present on arterial blood gas but is also nonspecific. The CXR is abnormal in the majority of patients who have PE with infarction, but these findings are often nonspecific. These findings may include infiltrates, atelectasis, and pleural effusion. More specific radiographic signs include Westermark's and Hampton's sign, although they are uncommon. Westermark's sign is the loss of pulmonary markings distal to the PE, from dilated pulmonary vasculature proximal to the embolus, with oligemia distally. Hampton's "hump" is pleural-based wedge-shaped opacity facing the hilum.

The electrocardiogram is also often abnormal and nonspecific. Sinus tachycardia and nonspecific ST-T wave changes are the most common abnormalities. Signs of right-sided heart strain, such as $S_1Q_3T_3$, T-wave inversion in leads V_1 to V_3, and a new right bundle branch block, are specific but uncommon [20]. Echocardiography is used to assess for signs of right heart strain and to look for thrombus in the right ventricle. Signs of pulmonary hypertension may include increased pressure over the tricuspid valve and the pulmonary artery. The definitive tests are ventilation perfusion imaging, multidetector pulmonary CT angiography, and, in rare circumstances, pulmonary angiography. Any patient who requires this type of examination should be transferred to the hospital to rule out the diagnosis.

Management

The definitive diagnosis cannot be made in most outpatient facilities, thus rapid transfer to a hospital is crucial to effective management. Patients who appear to be in acute distress should have only their airway, breathing, and circulation examined before transfer measures have begun. Those who appear to be in no acute distress may undergo a more detailed examination. Patients in acute distress should have an IV line started, placed on oxygen, and put on a cardio-pulmonary monitor.

After the history and physical have been completed, the physician should designate the patient's pretest probability for having a PE. The probability may be low, intermediate, or high, although there is no standard method for measurement of pretest probability. Some researchers have based this on objective data not available in the outpatient environment. The outpatient designation should reflect findings on history, examination, and other objective data. This pretest probability can be relayed to the admitting physician as a means to assist in determining what diagnostic test to perform. If the patient is believed to be at high risk for a PE and has no contraindications for anticoagulation, then heparin administration should be considered. From the outpatient view, the most important management point is to immediately transfer any patient suspected of having a PE (see Table 3).

Asthma

Asthma is characterized by reversible airflow obstruction, bronchial hyperresponsiveness, airway inflammation, submucosal edema, and increased mucus production caused by hypertrophy and hyperplasia of goblet cells [22–24]. Asthma is the most common chronic lung disease in developed and developing countries, with a current adult prevalence of 5%, and has been increasing in prevalence over the last 20 years [25,26]. It is also the most common cause of respiratory emergency, resulting in almost 2 million ED visits each year, 10% to 20% of which require hospital admission [22–28]. Between 4% and 10% of asthma admissions will require care in the ICU, but the presentations of severe acute asthma requiring ICU care have decreased over the last decade [26–28]. Although the death rate caused by asthma is low, 0.3 per 100,000 people, it is still responsible for approximately 5500 deaths per year, with the overwhelming majority of these patients suffering respiratory arrest before arriving at the hospital [25,27].

History

During an exacerbation, patients commonly report dyspnea, wheezing, tightness in the chest, and coughing (usually nonproductive). Frequent causes include viral respiratory infections, bacterial infections (most commonly by *Mycoplasma pneumoniae* and *Chlamydia pneumoniae*), exposure to allergens or respiratory irritants (tobacco smoke, perfumes, and fumes from cleaning products), exercise, exposure to cold, emotional distress, medications (aspirin, nonsteroidal anti-inflammatory drugs, or β-blockers), and noncompliance to medication [22–24,29]. Risk factors for increased morbidity and mortality include two or more ED visits or a hospital admission within the past year, any previous episode requiring mechanical ventilation, chronic steroid use, extremely rapid onset of symptoms, association of anaphylaxis, low socioeconomic and educational status, psychosocial disorders, and language barriers [22–24,29]. A large proportion of the asthma fatalities that occur are believed to be caused by extensive mucous plugging of the airways, with such air trapping that the lungs remain inflated at autopsy after removal from the thorax [22–24]. The failure of the patient or physician to recognize the severity of the asthma attack is also believed to be responsible for many of the deaths [25,30].

Physical examination

Asthma, meaning "panting" in Greek, was described accurately in ancient times for the most obvious clinical feature: tachypnea [22]. Wheezing is often heard diffusely and may be appreciated throughout the respiratory cycle or more prominently with expiration. Because airflow is required to cause turbulence, which produces wheezing, a patient with severe airway obstruction may have minimal airflow and therefore no wheezing. A brief, focused history and physical examination should be performed initially to identify any patient who may be unstable or need immediate airway interventions or assisted ventilation. An initial peak expiratory flow rate (PEFR) should be obtained. A focused examination, including vital signs, mental status, cardiopulmonary examination, and PEFR should be repeated frequently and after interventions to assess response to treatment.

A patient with only a mild exacerbation, defined as an initial PEFR ≥ 200 L/min or $\geq 50\%$ of the predicted best may have only end-expiratory wheezing and a slightly increased respiratory rate without other physical findings. During a moderate asthma exacerbation, a PEFR of 80 to 200 L/min or 25% to 50% of the predicted best, the patient may not be able to speak conversationally without breathlessness, they may not be able to recline on the stretcher and instead choose a more upright posture, respiratory rate will be increased, and wheezing will be more prominent. With a severe exacerbation, a PEFR of ≤ 80 L/min or $\leq 25\%$ of the predicted best, the patient will likely have diaphoresis, supraclavicular retractions, accessory muscle use, halting speech, a tripodding posture (sitting or standing while leaning forward to brace the arms outward on the knees or a fixed object), and severe tachypnea. Beware of agitation or confusion, cyanosis, fatigue, or a quiet chest because these are signs of impending respiratory arrest [22–24,29,30]. An increased pulsus paradoxus, ≥ 25 mm Hg, may be found with severe asthmatic exacerbations. Because this abnormality depends on forceful inspiratory and expiratory excursions, the pulsus may diminish as the clinical condition improves, airway obstruction resolves, and respiratory effort normalizes or as the condition worsens and the respiratory effort becomes fatiguing [22–28].

Diagnostic studies

In addition to the assessment of PEFR and oxygen saturation, the physician should consider obtaining a chest radiograph if the patient has not responded adequately to therapy or is in extremis. The film findings may be normal or may show signs of air trapping (increased lung volumes and flattened diaphragms). The actual value of the chest radiograph is to determine whether other serious complications, such as a pneumothorax or pulmonary infiltrate, may also be involved. Laboratory tests, if any, should be ordered specifically to each individual patient. One should consider checking electrolyte levels if the patient is given frequent or continuous β-agonist treatments or if underlying deficiencies of potassium, magnesium, or phosphate are suspected because this therapy will cause an intracellular shift of these ions, thereby further reducing serum levels [25]. Arterial blood gas (ABG) analysis may be performed to confirm a respiratory alkalosis condition caused by tachypnea or follow the resolution of hypercapnea once mechanical ventilation has been instituted, but it should be stressed that the need for an artificial airway and assisted ventilation is based on clinical assessments and must not be delayed while waiting for ABG or other diagnostic results [28].

Management

Oxygen should be administered to keep the arterial oxygen saturation (SaO_2) at $\geq 90\%$ and $\geq 95\%$ in pregnant patients or those who have significant CAD [25]. Inhaled β-agonists are the first-line therapy in all asthma exacerbations. They may be delivered with equivalent success by nebulization or by metered-dose-inhaler (MDI) with or without a spacer device [26–28]. A typical nebulized dose of albuterol would be 5 mg every 15 to 20 minutes times three doses. A similar effect can be obtained by giving a continuous nebulized treatment of 15 to 20 mg of albuterol over 1 hour. If a MDI is used, 6 to 8 actuations, 90 μg each, should be given at each treatment to deliver an equivalent dose [26,27,30]. Levalbuterol, the all R-isomer of albuterol (as opposed to the equal mixture of R and S in the standard racemic albuterol) has been shown to be as safe and effective at a dose of 1.25 mg per nebulized treatment and may even be more effective in certain subsets of asthmatics [25]. Ipratropium bromide should also be administered, either by nebulized treatment, 500 μg, or by 4 to 6 MDI actuations. Parenteral β-agonists should be used only if the patient is moribund, coughing excessively, or continues to worsen despite inhaled treatments [26,27,30]. The indicated dosage for epinephrine is 0.2 to 0.5 mg subcutaneously of a 1:1000 solution for three doses every 20 to 30 minutes. If the patient is in shock, it should be given as an IV bolus of 0.2 to 0.5 mg of 1:10,000 solution, followed by an infusion titrated between 1 and 20 μg/min. An alternative option for the subcutaneous route is terbutaline, 0.25 mg every 20 minutes for three doses [25,28].

Glucocorticoid steroid administration has been shown to decrease admission rates and prevent relapses and should be given to the majority of patients presenting with an asthmatic exacerbation. The one group that does not require steroids are those with very mild symptoms of short duration, which resolve completely with one inhaled bronchodilator, reflecting only bronchoconstriction without airway inflammation and edema [25,28]. The recommended oral dose of prednisone is 40 to 60 mg (0.5–1.0 mg/kg) daily for 3 to 14 days, with or without a taper. If the patient cannot tolerate the oral administration of prednisone, then methylprednisolone IV, 125 to 250 mg can be given [22–25,27,30].

Dehydration is common, especially if the exacerbation has been ongoing for several days, so that IV fluid administration is recommended by most experts for moderate to severe asthma attacks [3,27]. If an infiltrate is found on chest radiography or empiric antibiotics are given, coverage should include *Mycoplasma* and *Chlamydia* spp [1]. In severe exacerbations, the IV rapid infusion of magnesium sulfate, 2 g over 10 to 20 minutes, has been found to give additional clinical benefit [3,14,16]. There may be some role for the initiation of inhaled steroids or oral leukotriene antagonists in acute exacerbations, but more data need to be collected before these agents can be recommended without reservations [25,26,28]. A mixture of helium and oxygen (heliox) has been found to decrease the work of breathing and improve oxygenation in severe attacks by decreasing airway turbulence and resistance. To be effective, the formulation needs to be 70% to 80% helium and the remainder oxygen, so that heliox is not indicated if the patient requires high oxygen concentrations to maintain an adequate SaO_2 [25,28]. There is no role for sedatives, mucolytics, or opiate cough suppressants in the treatment of acute asthma [25,27].

Most patients will improve after treatments, with only 20% of all asthmatics ever requiring hospitalization [28]. Patients presenting with a PEFR $\leq 25\%$ of their predicted rate before treatment will likely require admission; if their PEFR remains below 25% despite aggressive therapy, then an ICU stay is warranted. If they improve but PEFR is still $\leq 40\%$, then admission is also indicated. Patients who show improvement but not resolution of their symptoms and a PEFR from 40% to 60% should be observed in the office or sent to the emergency department for continued treatment; after an additional 2 to 3 hours, if they have improved, then they can be sent home; but if not, then they should be admitted. Patients who reach a PEFR $\geq 60\%$ of their predicted best will most likely experience a resolution of subjective symptoms and can be sent home [2,28]. Given the mortality rate associated with asthma, any patient who does not respond to outpatient therapy should be considered for emergency department care to help determine the best course of therapy and to help determine disposition.

Chronic obstructive pulmonary disease

COPD encompasses a group of chronic lung disorders, but emphysema and chronic bronchitis are the disorders most commonly encountered in clinical practice and will be the focus of this discussion. A reduction in bronchial airflow caused by nonreversible disorders is the underlying pathophysiology. Permanent enlargement of air spaces distal to the terminal bronchiole with wall destruction but without fibrosis defines emphysema. The loss of elastic recoil of lung tissue allows the collapse of distal airways, promoting air trapping [1]. COPD has an incidence of 34.1 per 1000 people over the age 65 years, affecting 14 to 20 million people in the United States, making it the fourth leading cause of death [27,31]. It is responsible for 4 million office visits and 500,000 hospital admissions yearly. COPD patients typically experience one to three exacerbations per year, in which between 3% and 16% of the episodes require hospitalization; the mortality rate is 3% to 10% for each hospital stay [31].

History

The typical baseline symptoms of COPD patients include dyspnea and chronic cough with sputum production. During an exacerbation, the dyspnea will worsen, with an increase in tachypnea, a prolonged expiratory phase, and audible wheezing, and the sputum will often increase in volume while becoming purulent [22–24,31]. Approximately 80% of COPD exacerbations are believed to be caused by respiratory infections, with half being viral and half being bacterial [22–24]. Pulmonary irritants (cigarette smoke, smog, and ozone) and medication noncompliance are also common causes. The four elements responsible for the reduction in airflow during an exacerbation are mucosal edema, increased secretions, bronchial smooth muscle constriction, and airway inflammation [22–24].

Physical examination

COPD patients presenting with an acute exacerbation typically have an increased respiratory and heart rate and pursed-lip breathing with a prolonged expiratory phase of the respiratory cycle. The patient's thorax is often increased in the anteroposterior dimension to accommodate the increased lung volumes. Patients will position themselves to maximize respiratory mechanics, often bracing their hands on their knees to stabilize the upper extremities and recruit accessory muscles. An examination of their lungs may reveal expiratory wheezing or may simply be quiet, with markedly diminished air exchange. Other life-threatening disorders that are associated with COPD should be considered, such as pneumothorax, which may produce asymmetric or absent breath sounds on a hemithorax, distended neck veins, and tracheal deviation, whereas pneumonia may cause signs of focal pulmonary consolidation or pleural effusion. Acute agitation may be a sign of hypoxemia, whereas somnolence or lethargy may indicate an elevated partial pressure of carbon dioxide (PcO_2) caused by hypercarbic respiratory insufficiency.

Diagnostic studies

Continuous pulse oximetry is necessary to ensure an adequate level of SaO_2 ($\geq 88\%$–90%), especially if supplemental oxygen is being administered, without overshooting and encouraging CO_2 retention by suppression of the hypoxic respiratory drive [22–24]. Chest radiographs typically reveal hyperinflation with flattened diaphragms and may also show bullae and pulmonary oligemia [22–24]. During a presumed COPD exacerbation, the additional value of the CXR is to evaluate for other causes of acute dyspnea, including pneumothorax, pneumonia, and congestive heart failure. Between 16% and 21% of COPD patients have CXR findings that were believed to be helpful by physicians, and treatments were then modified by the findings [31]. Serum electrolytes may be indicated to determine potassium and phosphate level because these are commonly depleted in COPD patients, and serum levels may drop further from intracellular shifts induced by β-agonists. ABG analysis, if available urgently, may be particularly helpful to evaluate for acute CO_2 retention indicated by an elevated PcO_2 with an acidosis. Although they are not commonly performed at the time of an exacerbation, if pulmonary function tests (PFTs) are obtained, they will confirm an obstructive pattern: a decreased ratio of forced expiratory volume in 1 second (FEV_1)/forced vital capacity (FVC), an increased total lung capacity and residual volume, and decreased diffusing capacity [22–24].

Management

Oxygen administration is recommended to keep the SaO2 level at $\geq 88\%$ to 90% and the PO_2 at ≥ 60 mm Hg to maintain tissue oxygenation while preventing pulmonary vasoconstriction and right ventricular strain or pressure overload [22–24,31]. Inhaled β-agonists and anticholinergics should be given by nebulizer or MDI. Albuterol and ipratropium are the most common representatives of these respective classes in the United States. Their effects are additive, so they should be used together, and although albuterol will often give muscular tremor and tachycardia, ipratropium rarely produces any significant side effects [22–24]. Theophylline has been in use for over 70 years and has been found to improve FEV_1 and exercise performance by about 10% in COPD patients by increasing diaphragm strength and endurance and mucociliary clearance. Because theophylline has a narrow therapeutic index, the associated side effects of nausea, vomiting, and tremor are common, whereas life-threatening toxicity includes seizures and cardiac arrhythmias. For these reasons, theophylline has little role acutely but may have a role in outpatient chronic care if used cautiously [22–24,27].

Glucocortical steroids are beneficial acutely and improve outcomes in COPD exacerbations. Either a short course, 4 to 7 days without taper, or a 10- to 14-day course with a taper is effective. Prednisone, 0.5 to 1 mg/kg orally each day, can be used, but an initial dose of IV methylprednisolone or dexamethasone can be given if patients are unable to tolerate oral medications. There is currently not enough evidence to recommend initiating inhaled steroids for acute COPD episodes, but they may also prove to be helpful [22–24,27,31]. Prescribing antibiotics for an exacerbation is believed to decrease bacterial counts in the chronically colonized respiratory tracts of COPD patients. Currently, the agents recommended for 7- to 10-day outpatient therapy include trimethoprim-sulfamethoxazole, ampicillin, doxycycline, and erythromycin. If the patient has an infiltrate on CXR or has fever or signs of systemic infection, then IV antibiotics effective against *Streptococcus pneumoniae* and *Haemophilus influenzae* should be started [22–24]. Expectorants and mucolytics have been found to provide little or no benefit [22–24,27].

Noninvasive positive pressure ventilation, using either continuous positive airway pressure or bi-level positive airway pressure, may decrease the work of breathing and improve ventilation, but patient cooperation is required to be effective. If acute respiratory failure occurs with hypoxemia ($PO_2 \leq 50$ mm Hg) and respiratory acidosis despite aggressive medical therapy, tracheal intubation and mechanical ventilation are indicated. These patients should be ventilated cautiously because overzealous correction of acute or chronic hypercarbia may cause severe alkalemia, precipitating seizures or ventricular arrhythmias [22–24].

The majority of COPD patients will improve after therapy and can safely return home. Patients who continue to have dyspnea increased over their baseline will need to be hospitalized if they also experience an inability to walk (if previously ambulatory), loss of appetite or sleep caused by dyspnea, comorbid pulmonary (eg, pneumonia) or nonpulmonary (eg, anemia) conditions, worsened hypoxemia or hypercarbia, new or worsened cor pulmonale, and an inability to manage at home with health care resources (eg, home oxygen) not readily available. Patients will need to be admitted to an ICU if they have alterations in mental status (confusion or lethargy), respiratory fatigue, worsening hypoxemia despite supplemental oxygen, worsening respiratory acidosis (pH ≤ 7.30), and the need for mechanical ventilation (invasive or noninvasive) [31].

Pneumonia

Pneumonia is inflammation, most often from infection, affecting the lung parenchyma (respiratory bronchioles and alveolar units) [22–24]. Although there are multiple distinct causes, including viral, fungal, and mycobacterial pneumonias, aspiration pneumonia, ventilator or hospital-acquired pneumonia, and opportunistic infections in immunodeficient individuals, this discussion focuses on community-acquired bacterial pneumonia in immunocompetent adults. An infectious agent is identified in 30% to 40% of the cases of community-acquired pneumonia (CAP), in which the most common bacterial organism is *S pneumoniae*, followed by *C pneumoniae*, *M pneumoniae*, and *H influenzae*. *Legionella pneumonia* is a rare causative agent in the very elderly (1% in those ≥ 80 years old) but is more common in younger adults (8% in those ≤ 80 years old). Gram-negative enteric organisms are more common in older patients who have comorbid conditions, particularly diabetes, malignancy, central nervous system disease, and renal, hepatic, or cardiopulmonary diseases [32–34].

The incidence of pneumonia in the United States is 12 cases per 1000 patients per year, resulting in 4 to 5.6 million cases annually. Approximately 25% of these patients will require hospitalization, and 10% of those will require an ICU stay. The risk for developing pneumonia is 10-fold higher in residents of long-term care facilities than for older adults living in the community [27,29,32,35,36]. Pneumonia is the leading cause of infectious deaths and the sixth overall cause of mortality in the United States; in people over age 65, pneumonia moves up to the fifth leading cause of death, resulting in 60 thousand deaths per year. The mortality rate for pneumonia varies depending on the location of treatment, which is a marker for the severity of the disease. For those treated as outpatients, the rate is very low, between ≤1% and 9%, but it is higher for inpatients and approaches 50% in an ICU [32,36,37].

History

Cough, purulent sputum, dyspnea, and pleuritic thoracic pain are reported commonly, localizing symptoms associated with pneumonia; nonspecific symptoms include fever and chills, headache, and myalgias. Elderly patients may have fewer of these symptoms and are more likely than are younger adults to present with a change in mental status. If the lower lobes of the lungs are involved, diaphragmatic irritation can cause upper abdominal pain, referred shoulder or scapular pain, or singultus [32,37,38].

Physical examination

Fever, increased heart rate and respiratory rate, inspiratory crackles, and signs of consolidation (bronchial breath sounds, egophony, increased tactile fremitus) on lung examination are found typically. The patient may appear fatigued, but a rapid evaluation of the mental status is vital to evaluate for possible impending respiratory failure. The skin, mucous membranes, and jugular veins should be examined for evidence of dehydration. Abdominal distension and diminished bowel sounds may be found, caused by paralytic ileus, particularly with lower-lobe pneumonia. SaO_2 may also be decreased, requiring supplemental oxygen to maintain normal values [37,38].

Diagnostic studies

Chest radiography is necessary to confirm the presence and location of the pneumonia. It may show focal consolidation of air-space pneumonia or a diffuse interstitial pattern; it is also helpful in evaluating for other conditions that may present similarly, such as CHF of a neoplasm. A leukocytosis with an increased percentage of PMNs and immature band forms is common, but leukopenia may occur. ABG analysis, if available, may reveal respiratory acidosis and an elevated PaO_2/FIO_2 ratio, showing evidence of respiratory failure caused by severe pneumonia [37,38]. The Infectious

Disease Society of America [34] recommends obtaining a sputum specimen for Gram staining and culture on all inpatients treated for pneumonia, whereas the American Thoracic Society recommends ordering a specimen only if an organism is suspected to be drug resistant or not susceptible to the usual empiric therapy. Blood cultures yield low results and may not need to be ordered routinely, based on studies showing that there were no significant differences in culture rates among patients who have differing pneumonia severity scores and that the rates of bacteremia in pneumonia patients did not significantly influence their hospital stay or mortality rate. Furthermore, blood culture results only rarely offer guidance for clinical decisions or changes in therapy [34,37,39]. A new urinary antigen assay for S pneumoniae, which has an 82% sensitivity for diagnosing bacteremia, is now available and may be helpful in identifying these patients [40].

Management

Most patients diagnosed with pneumonia can be treated with oral antibiotics, but an IV dose should be administered if the patient is unable to take medications orally or is suspected to be bacteremic or acutely ill. The current recommendation by the American Infectious Disease Society of America for the treatment of CAP in adults is a second- or third-generation cephalosporin plus a macrolide or an extended spectrum fluoroquinolone. If the patient is admitted to an ICU, broad-spectrum antibiotics are indicated and should include coverage for *Pseudomonas* organisms if risk factors are present (bronchiectasis, chronic steroid therapy, or recent antibiotic administration) [27,35,37,40,41]. The early initiation of antibiotics (within 8 hours of the patient's arrival) has been shown to decrease the length of stay in the hospital and reduce inpatient and 30-day mortality in patients older than 65 years. The optimum duration of antibiotic therapy is not well defined but is typically from 7 to 21 days [27,35,37,41,42]. Supplemental oxygen should be supplied to maintain a normal SaO_2, and IV fluids should be administered if the patient has signs of significant dehydration.

Numerous grading systems and scoring scales have been created in an attempt to predict which patients are at higher risk for complications and mortality and require hospitalization or even an ICU stay versus those patients at low risk who can be safely treated as outpatients. Some of these systems include the Pneumonia Severity Index, the Pneumonia Outcome Research Trial (PORT), the British Thoracic Society Scoring System, and the American Thoracic Society Criteria for Severe CAP. These scoring systems generally include similar data (vital signs, comorbidities, CXR, and laboratory studies) to separate patients into different risk classes. Patients are considered to be at high risk and should be hospitalized if they have any of the following: age ≥ 65 years, respiratory rate ≥ 30 breaths/min, bilateral or multilobar infiltrates, hypotension (systolic ≤ 90 mm Hg, diastolic ≤ 60 mm Hg), acute renal failure, and altered mental status. If the patient has respiratory failure (defined by PaO_2/FIO_2 ratio ≥ 250 or the need for mechanical ventilation) or is in septic shock requiring vasopressors, then ICU care will certainly be required. The study result of concern, however, is that in one review of patients in the ICU for CAP, 11% had Pneumonia Severity Index class I scores, and 13% had class II scores (I–V, with I least and V most severe) [35–38,41,43].

Miscellaneous disorders

Many other less prevalent disorders may lead to dyspnea, some of which can be life threatening and require immediate treatment, whereas others are subacute or chronic conditions for which patients may be followed and treated as outpatients. The history and physical examination often assist in diagnosing these entities, but there may be a need for diagnostic studies (chest radiograph, laboratory studies, referral for pulmonary function studies, laryngoscopy, or bronchoscopy).

Spontaneous pneumothorax can occur without trauma or iatrogenic lung injury and can be further divided into primary (young patients who have normal lung parenchyma but congenital apical blebs) and secondary (older patients who have underlying lung disease such as emphysema or pulmonary fibrosis). The risk is higher for smokers and is greater for men than women. Pleuritic chest pain and dyspnea are the most common complaints. Diminished or asymmetric breath sounds over the affected hemithorax are found on examination. A CXR, specifically an upright expiratory film, is the confirmatory test. Chest tube thoracostomy placement or anterior needle decompression should be performed emergently if the patient appears to have a tension pneumothorax (distended neck veins, tracheal deviation to the opposite side, and hypotension). For small, stable pneumothoracies, simple aspiration is effective but takes longer until resolution than the tube thoracostomy does [27]. These therapies will in most cases require transfer to the ED.

Airway obstruction may be organic, occurring as a result of laryngeal tumors, polyps, or vocal cord paralysis, or be caused by functional vocal cord disorders, such as paradoxical vocal cord movement. Dyspnea and stridor are common features, and visualization of the glottis may be needed to diagnose the obstruction [1,44]. Patients who have neuromuscular diseases resulting in acute weakness, such as Guillain-Barré syndrome or myasthenia gravis, will report dyspnea because they may be using a much greater percentage of their respiratory strength than previously to accomplish thoracic expansion and diaphragmatic excursion. Anxiety disorders often have dyspnea as a central complaint, and hyperventilation syndrome may be identified. Patients who have COPD have a 3-fold increase in the prevalence of anxiety disorders than the general population, so that it may be difficult to readily make this diagnosis [45].

Central nervous system events such as strokes or intracranial hemorrhages will often cause tachypnea and a resultant respiratory alkalosis, but dyspnea is not usually reported [46]. Liver disease and pregnancy are also associated with an increase in minute ventilation. Moderate to severe anemia will typically cause dyspnea on exertion because of reduced oxygen delivery to peripheral tissues. Metabolic acidosis of any cause (sepsis, increased lactate, or diabetic or alcoholic ketosis) will cause a compensatory increase in minute ventilation that is sensed as SOB by the patient. Toxins, including carbon monoxide and salicylate poisoning, will also cause a symptomatic increase in respiratory rate and tidal volume. These patients, unless a secondary disorder is involved, will all show normal findings on lung examinations.

Summary

When evaluating a dyspneic patient in the office, a quick initial assessment of the airway, breathing, and circulation, while gathering a brief history and focused physical examination are necessary. Most often, an acute cardiopulmonary disorder, such as CHF, cardiac ischemia, pneumonia, asthma, or COPD exacerbation, can be identified and treated. Stable patients who improve can be sent home, but those in acute distress with unstable or impending unstable conditions need to be transferred emergently to definitive care. Because of the difficult logistics involved in attempting to work up an outpatient for new onset of SOB, some patients will need to be transferred to the nearest ED for a definitive diagnosis.

Further readings

Shilon Y, Shitrit AB-G, Rudensky B, et al. A rapid quantitative D-dimer assay at admission correlates with the severity of community acquired pneumonia. Blood Coagul Fibrinolysis 2003; 14(8):745–8.
Stein PD, Terrin ML, Hales CA, et al. Clinical, laboratory, roentgenographic and electrocardiographic findings in patients with acute pulmonary embolism and no pre-existing cardiac or pulmonary disease. Chest 1991;100:598.

References

[1] Zoorob RJ, Cambell JS. Acute dyspnea in the office. Am Fam Physician 2003;68:1803–10.
[2] Kunitoh H, Wantanabe K, Sajima Y. Clinical features to predict hypoxia and/or hypercapnea in acute asthma attacks. J Asthma 1994;31:401–7.
[3] Hazinski MF, Cummins RO, Field JM. 2000 Handbook of emergency cardiovascular care for healthcare providers. Dallas (TX): American Heart Association; 2000.
[4] Packer M, Cohn JN; for the Steering Committee and Membership of the Advisory Council to Improve Outcomes Nationwide in Heart Failure. Consensus recommendations for the management of chronic heart failure, II: management of heart failure: approaches to the prevention of heart failure. Am J Cardiol 1999;83(Suppl 2A):9A–38A.
[5] The Criteria Committee of the New York Heart Association. Physical capacity with heart disease. In: Diseases of the heart and blood vessels, nomenclature and criteria for diagnosis. 6th edition. Boston: Little, Brown & Co; 1964. p. 110–4.
[6] Cutaia M. Ambulatory monitoring of oxygen saturation in chronic lung disease: optimizing long-term oxygen therapy. Clinical Pulmonary Medicine 2002;9(6):297–305.

[7] McDonagh TA, Robb SD, Murdoch DR, et al. Biochemical detection of left-ventricular systolic dysfunction. Lancet 1998;351:9–13.

[8] Maisel AS, Koon J, Krishnaswamy P, et al. Utility of B-natriuretic peptide as a rapid, point-of-care test for screening patients undergoing echocardiography to determine left ventricular dysfunction. Am Heart J 2001;141:367–74.

[9] American Heart Association. Heart and stroke facts: 1995 statistical supplement. Dallas (TX): American Heart Association; 1994.

[10] Tucker NHB, Doty D, Gilmour K, et al, for the Early Diagnosis Steering Committee. Assessment and triage of unstable angina and acute MI. 1998.

[11] Canto JG, Every NR, Magid DJ, et al, for the National Registry of Myocardial Infarction 2 Investigators. The volume of primary angioplasty procedures and survival after acute myocardial infarction. N Engl J Med 2000;342:1573–80.

[12] Deedwania PC, Carbajal E. Silent myocardial ischemia: a clinical perspective. Arch Intern Med 1991;151:2373–82.

[13] Canto JG, Shlipak MG, Rogers WJ, et al. Prevalence, clinical characteristics, and mortality among patients with myocardial infarction presenting without chest pain. JAMA 2000;283: 3223.

[14] Yusuf S, Hawken S, Ounpuu S, et al. Effect of potentially modifiable risk factors associated with myocardial infarction in 52 countries (the INTERHEART study): case-control study. Lancet 2004;364:937.

[15] Antman EM, Anbe DT, Armstrong PW, et al. ACC/AHA guidelines for the management of patients with ST-elevation myocardial infarction–executive summary: a report of the American College of Cardiology/American Heart Association Task Force on Practice Guidelines (Writing Committee to Revise the 1999 Guidelines for the Management of Patients With Acute Myocardial Infarction). Circulation 2004;110:588.

[16] Parker JO. Nitrates and angina pectoris. Am J Cardiol 1993;72:3C–8C.

[17] Teo KK, Yusuf S, Furberg CD. Effects of prophylactic antiarrhythmic drug therapy in acute myocardial infarction: An overview of results from randomized controlled trials. JAMA 1993;270:1589.

[18] Calder KK, Herbert M, Henderson SO. The mortality of untreated pulmonary embolism in emergency department patients. Ann Emerg Med 2005;45:302–10.

[19] Fedullo PF, Tapson VF. The evaluation of suspected pulmonary embolism. N Engl J Med 2003;349:1247–56.

[20] Horlander KT, Mannino DM, Leeper KV. Pulmonary embolism mortality in the United States, 1979–1998: an analysis using multiple-cause mortality data. Arch Intern Med 2003; 163:1711.

[21] Investigators PIOPED. Value of the ventilation/perfusion scan in acute pulmonary embolism: results of the prospective investigation of pulmonary embolism diagnosis (PIOPED). JAMA 1990;263:2753–9.

[22] Adams L, Stulbarg MS. Dyspnea. In: Murray JF, Nadel JA, editors. Textbook of respiratory medicine. 3rd edition. Philadelphia: WB Saunders; 2000. p. 542–9.

[23] Rennard SI, Shapiro SD, Snider GL. COPD. In: Murray JF, Nadel JA, editors. Textbook of respiratory medicine. 3rd edition. Philadelphia: WB Saunders; 2000. p. 1188–230.

[24] Bushey HA, Burchard EG, Corry DB, et al. Asthma. In: Murray JF, Nadel JA, editors. Textbook of respiratory medicine. 3rd edition. Philadelphia: WB Saunders; 2000. p. 1250–77.

[25] Jaroslaw P, Nowak RM, Zoratti EM. The evaluation and management of acute, severe asthma. Med Clin North Am 2002;86:1049–71.

[26] Cates C, Fitzgerald M. Asthma. In: Clinical evidence. Vol. 4. London: BMJ Publishing Group; 2000. p. 828–64.

[27] Gibbs MA, Camargo CA, Rowe BH, et al. State of the art: therapeutic controversies in severe acute asthma. Acad Emerg Med 2000;7(7):800–15.

[28] Rodrigo GJ, Rodrigo C, Hall JB. Acute asthma in adults: a review. Chest 2004;125(3): 1081–102.

[29] Sherman S. Acute asthma in adults. In: Tintinalli J, Ruiz E, Krome RL, editors. Emergency medicine: a comprehensive study guide. 4th edition. New York: McGraw-Hill Co; 1996. p. 430–7.

[30] Beveridge RC, Grunfeld AF, Hodder RV, et al. Guidelines for the emergency management of asthma in adults. CMAJ 1996;155(1):25–37.

[31] Soto FJ, Varkey B. Evidence-based approach to acute exacerbations of COPD. Curr Opin Pulm Med 2003;9(2):117–24.

[32] Loeb M. Pneumonia in the elderly. Curr Opin Infect Dis 2004;17(2):127–30.

[33] Bjerre LM, Verheij TJM, Kochen MM. Antibiotics for community acquired pneumonia in adult outpatients. Cochrane Database Syst Rev 2004;3:CD002109.

[34] Garcia-Vazquez E, Marcos MA, Mensa J, et al. Assessment of the usefulness of sputum culture for diagnosis of community-acquired pneumonia using the PORT predictive scoring system. Arch Intern Med 2004;164(16):1807–11.

[35] Wilkinson M, Woodhead MA. Guidelines for community-acquired pneumonia in the ICU. Curr Opin Crit Care 2004;10(1):59–64.

[36] Riley PD, Aronsky D, Dean NC. Validation of the 2001 American Thoracic Society criteria for severe community-acquired pneumonia. Crit Care Med 2004;32(12):2398–402.

[37] Alves DW, Kennedy MT. Community-acquired pneumonia in casualty: etiology, clinical features, diagnosis, and management (or a look at the "new" in pneumonia since 2002). Curr Opin Pulm Med 2004;10(3):166–70.

[38] Metlay JP, Fine MJ. Testing strategies in the initial management of patients with community-acquired pneumonia. Ann Intern Med 2003;138(2):109–18.

[39] Ioachimescu OC, Ioachimescu AG, Iannini PB. Severity scoring in community-acquired pneumonia caused by *Streptococcus pneumoniae*: a 5-year experience. Int J Antimicrob Agents 2004;24(5):485–90.

[40] Battleman DS, Callahan M, Thaler HT. Rapid antibiotic delivery and appropriate antibiotic selection reduce length of hospital stay of patients with community-acquired pneumonia. Arch Intern Med 2002;162:682–8.

[41] Alvarez-Lerma F, Torres A. Severe community-acquired pneumonia. Current Opinion in Critical Care 2004;10(5):369–74.

[42] Silber SH, Garrett C, Singh R, et al. Early administration of antibiotics does not shorten time to clinical stability in patients with moderate-to-severe community-acquired pneumonia. Chest 2003;124(5):1798–804.

[43] Oosterheert JJ. Comparison of guidelines for diagnosis of severe community-acquired pneumonia. Curr Opin Infect Dis 2003;16(2):153–9.

[44] McGeehan M, Busse WW. Refractory asthma. Med Clin North Am 2002;86:1073–90.

[45] Brenes GA. Anxiety and chronic obstructive pulmonary disease: prevalence, impact, and treatment. Psychosom Med 2003;65(6):963–70.

[46] Rose BD, editor. Respiratory acidosis. In: Clinical physiology of acid-base electrolyte disorders. 4th edition. New York: McGraw-Hill Co; 1994. p. 540–603.

ELSEVIER
SAUNDERS

THE MEDICAL
CLINICS
OF NORTH AMERICA

Med Clin N Am 90 (2006) 481–503

Acute Abdominal Pain

Mark H. Flasar, MD*, Eric Goldberg, MD

*Division of Gastroenterology and Hepatology, Department of Medicine,
University of Maryland Medical Center, Baltimore, MD, USA*

Abdominal pain is a common complaint in all settings of medical practice. In the United States in 2002, abdominal pain was the chief complaint of over 7 million patients presenting to an emergency department (ED), accounting for 6.5% of all patient visits [1]. In primary care practices in 2002, abdominal pain was a complaint of more than 13.5 million patient visits, accounting for 1.5% of patient encounters [2]. In certain situations, abdominal pain may be a symptom of a severe, life-threatening disease process, whereas in other situations, it may be a symptom of a more benign underlying condition. This review provides a framework for understanding abdominal pain, so that practitioners may determine those patients who need a more expedited evaluation, and reviews the pathophysiologic mechanisms underlying abdominal pain. A general approach to the patient is outlined, and several causes of abdominal pain are considered in detail, focusing on the most severe and commonly encountered.

A general understanding of abdominal anatomy, physiology, and pathophysiology is vital when formulating a differential diagnosis for abdominal pain. In addition, it is important to understand how abdominal pain is generated and perceived by the patient. The abdominal viscera are innervated with nociceptive afferents within the mesentery, on peritoneal surfaces, and within the mucosa and muscularis of hollow organs. These afferents respond to both mechanical and chemical stimuli, producing sensations of dull, crampy, insidious pain. The principal mechanical stimulus is stretching, whereas a variety of chemical stimuli, including substance P, serotonin, prostaglandins, and H^+ ions, are perceived as noxious by visceral chemoreceptors [3]. Abdominal pain occurs in three broad patterns, visceral, parietal, and referred. Visceral nociception typically involves stretching and

---

* Corresponding author. Division of Gastroenterology and Hepatology, Department of Medicine, University of Maryland Medical Center, 22 South Greene Street, Baltimore, MD 21201.

E-mail address: mflasar@medicine.umaryland.edu (M.H. Flasar).

distension of the abdominal organs, but torsion and contraction also contribute. The pain is carried on slow-conducting C-fibers. Patients often describe pain of visceral origin as a dull ache. Visceral pain is often located at the midline because visceral innervation of abdominal organs is typically bilateral. Pain location corresponds to those dermatomes that match the innervation of the injured organ [3]. Generally, visceral pain from organs proximal to the ligament of Treitz (embryonic foregut), including the hepatobiliary organs and spleen, is felt in the epigastrum. Visceral pain from abdominal organs between the ligament of Treitz and the hepatic flexure of the colon (embryonic midgut) is felt in the periumbilical region. Visceral pain generated from organs distal to the hepatic flexure (embryonic hindgut) is perceived in the midline lower abdomen. Parietal pain is typically sharp and well localized, resulting from the direct irritation of the peritoneal lining. Parietal peritoneal afferents are A delta fibers with a rapid conduction velocity, which results in a sharp pain sensation similar to skin and muscle pain. Because parietal innervation is unilateral, lateralization of pain occurs [3]. Referred pain occurs when visceral afferents carrying stimuli from a diseased organ enter the spinal cord at the same level as somatic afferents from a remote anatomic location; it is typically well localized. A single diseased organ may produce all three types of pain. For example, when a patient develops cholecystitis, gallbladder inflammation is experienced initially as a visceral pain in the epigastric region. Eventually, the inflammation extends to the parietal peritoneum, and the patient will experience parietal pain that lateralizes to the right upper quadrant. Gallbladder pain may also refer to the right shoulder.

Awareness of the anatomy and innervation of the abdominal viscera allows one to formulate a differential diagnosis of abdominal pain based on the location of the pain (Box 1). However, there is a significant overlap among abdominal pain presentations. Furthermore, disease processes from organs outside of the abdominal cavity can present with abdominal pain. To considerably narrow the differential diagnosis, it is crucial to approach each patient in a systematic, logical, and deliberate manner. Similar to the way in which physicians are trained to read an ECG by assessing rate, rhythm, axis, and other findings, so too should physicians approach abdominal pain. In an age of expanding variety, quality, and accuracy of diagnostic tests, abdominal pain also necessitates a regimented approach, which starts with a thorough history. William Osler stated, "By the historical method alone can many problems in medicine be approached profitably". The history should include not only a thorough assessment of the present condition but also a thorough assessment of underlying medical problems, medications, family history, and a history of substance abuse, recent travel, and occupation. Important clues to the cause of the pain should be determined in the patient's history by inquiring about the nature of the pain, which includes its quality, location, rapidity of onset, chronicity, radiation, intensity, exacerbating factors, alleviating factors, and associated symptoms.

After a thorough history, a focused physical examination should be performed. Quoting Osler again, "Don't touch the patient—state first what you see; cultivate your powers of observation". For example, a patient who has peritonitis often lies completely still because movement further irritates the peritoneum. On the other hand, a patient who has renal colic may writhe in pain and may not be able to be consoled to comfort. Once an initial observation is complete, a review of the vital signs is imperative. Any abnormality of vital signs should prompt the physician to consider the presence of an abdominal catastrophe. Auscultation of the abdomen determines whether the intestinal peristalsis is appropriate and whether any abdominal bruits are present. Next, palpation of the abdomen should be performed to distinguish pain, a subjective sensation, from tenderness, which is an objective finding. When performing palpation, the location of tenderness should be used to narrow the differential diagnosis. Additionally, the presence of guarding or rebound tenderness should be noted because these findings imply peritoneal irritation. Furthermore, palpation can determine the presence of visceral enlargement, masses, or fluid.

The importance of a properly executed history and physical examination cannot be overstated. Although the sensitivity and specificity of a history and physical may not match that of an abdominal CT scan, there is no risk, minimal time lost, and essentially no cost. In fact, in this evidence-based era, one observational study has revealed that, based on history and a physical alone, physicians were able to correctly differentiate between organic and nonorganic causes of abdominal pain nearly 80% of the time [4]. Furthermore, historical features such as pain location have been shown in prospective investigation to be specific for certain disease states [5]. That being stated, however, some of the basic physical examination tools have come under close scrutiny when assessed independently. For example, some studies suggest that the digital rectal examination fails to alter diagnosis or management, and routine performance may not be necessary [6]. However, the present authors believe that performing the rectal examination is crucial to the evaluation of acute abdominal pain. For example, the presence of occult blood in a patient's stool may suggest the presence of luminal ischemia in the appropriate clinical setting. Additionally, rectal tenderness can be seen with anal fissures, perirectal abscesses, or acute prostatitis. Thus, although the rectal examination may lack sensitivity or specificity, it can often help bring added focus to a blurry clinical presentation.

The ability to detect warning signs of impending disaster in a patient who presents with abdominal pain is often left up to the primary physician, long before the ED physician, surgeon, gastroenterologist, or other specialist encounters the patient. Certain historical and examination findings should raise "red flags" that a severe life-threatening underlying abdominal process is present and prompt early triage to an emergency department or inpatient hospital bed. Red flags from the history include fever, vomiting, obstipation, light-headedness, syncope, and overt gastrointestinal blood loss. Red flags

Box 1. Anatomic origin of pain

Right upper quadrant
Peptic ulcer disease
Biliary disease
  Biliary colic
  Cholecystititis
  Choledocholithiasis,
  Cholecystitis
  Cholangitis
Liver disease
  Hepatitis
  Neoplasm
  Abscess
  Congestive
  hepatopathy
Lung disease
  Pneumonia
  Subphrenic abscess
  Pulmonary embolism
  Pneumothorax
Abdominal wall
  Herpes Zoster
  Muscular stain
Kidney disease
  Pyelonephritis
  Perinephric abscess
  Nephrolithiasis
Colonic causes
  Colitis
  Right-sided
  diverticulitis

Middle upper abdomen
Peptic ulcer disease
Pancreatitic disease
  Pancreatitis
  Pancreatic neoplasm
Biliary disease
  Biliary colic
  Cholecystititis
  Choledocholithiasis
  Cholecystitis
  Cholangitis
Esophageal disease
  Reflux esophagitis
  Infectious esophagitis
  Pill esophagitis
Cardiac disease
  Myocardial ischemia
  or infarction
  Pericarditis
Abdominal aortic
aneurysm (AAA)
rupture/dissection

Mesenteric ischemia

Left upper quadrant
Peptic ulcer disease
Splenic disease
  Splenic rupture
  Splenic infarct
Pancreatic disease
  Pancreatitits
  Pancreatic neoplasm
Lung disease
  Pneumonia
  Subphrenic abscess
  Pulmonary embolism
  Pneumothorax
Kidney disease
  Pyelonephritis
  Perinephric abscess
  Nephrolithiasis

Periumbilical
Appendicitis (early)
Small bowel
obstruction
Gastroenteritis
Mesenteric ischemia
AAA rupture
AAA dissection

Right lower quadrant
Appendicitis
Inflammatory bowel
disease (IBD)
OB-GYN causes
  Ovarian tumor
  Ovarian torsion
  Ectopic pregnancy
  Pelvic inflammatory
  disease (PID)
  Tubo-ovarian abscess
Kidney disease
  Pyelonephritis
  Perinephric abscess
  Nephrolithiasis
Intestinal disease
  Right-sided
  diverticulitis
  Ileocolitis
  Gastroenteritis
  Hernia

Suprapubic
IBD
OB-GYN causes
  Ovarian tumor
  Ovarian torsion
  Ectopic pregnancy
  PID
  Tubo-ovarian abscess
  Dysmenorrhea
Colonic disease
  Proctocolitis
  Diverticulitis
Urinary tract disease
  Cystitis
  Nephrolithiasis
  Prostatitis

Left lower quadrant
IBD
OB-GYN causes
  Ovarian tumor
  Ovarian torsion
  Ectopic pregnancy
  PID
  Tubo-ovarian abscess
Kidney disease
  Pyelonephritis
  Perinephric abscess
  Nephrolithiasis
Intestinal disease
  Sigmoid diverticulitis
  Ileocolitis
  Gastroenteritis
  Hernia

Diffuse
Gastroenteritis
Bowel obstruction
Peritonitis
Mesenteric ischemia
IBD
Diabetic ketoacidosis
Porphyria
Uremia
Hypercalcemia
Sickle cell crisis
Vasculitis
Heavy metal
intoxication
Opiate withdrawl
Familial
Mediterranean fever
Hereditary angioedema

from the physical examination include any abnormality of the vital signs, mental status changes, involuntary guarding, rebound tenderness, the complete absence of bowel sounds, and pain out of proportion to the physical examination.

Although cardiac, pulmonary, urologic, musculoskeletal, and gynecologic causes of abdominal pain will not be specifically addressed in this article, it is imperative to keep these extra-abdominal disease processes in the differential diagnosis of abdominal pain. Red-flag indications that a life-threatening extra-abdominal cause of abdominal pain is present include chest pain, back pain, shortness of breath, vaginal bleeding, and hemodynamic instability. Finally, there are a multitude of systemic medical disorders, such as adrenal insufficiency, diabetic ketoacidosis, porphyria, and sickle cell pain crisis, that can present with abdominal pain. Evidence of these disorders in the patient's medical history, medications, or physical examination should prompt their consideration as the cause of the patient's pain.

The selection of imaging studies to evaluate abdominal pain should be guided by the differential diagnoses generated from the initial evaluation. Historically, plain abdominal radiographs have been the first imaging modality chosen for abdominal pain. They can be obtained rapidly and at a relatively low cost. However, with the evolution of more sensitive and specific modalities such as CT and ultrasonography, the value of the plain abdominal radiographic series has been debated. Nonetheless, plain films should be the initial imaging modality in patients who are suspected of having visceral perforation, obstruction, or foreign body ingestion or insertion.

The abdominal plain film series should include supine and upright abdominal films in conjunction with an upright chest (or lateral decubitus abdominal) film. Plain abdominal imaging has been estimated to be diagnostic in up to 60% of cases of suspected small bowel obstruction [7], although sensitivity is more limited in cases of low-grade obstruction [8]. The location, volume, and distribution of intraluminal air, the presence and distribution of air–fluid levels, and the luminal diameter can often be helpful in differentiating between an obstructive and nonobstructive process, such as a partial or complete large or small bowel obstruction, ileus, pseudo-obstruction, or a normal variant. Unfortunately, overlap in the radiographic appearance of obstructive and nonobstructive processes limits the sensitivity and specificity of plain films in this setting.

The ability of plain films to detect free air depends on the volume of free air within the peritoneal cavity. For the detection of large volumes, as would be expected with a perforated viscus, the sensitivity of plain films is reported to be as high as 100%. Sensitivity is maximized if the patient is placed in the upright or decubitus position for 5 to 10 minutes before obtaining an upright chest or lateral decubitus film, thereby allowing small volumes of air to redistribute to and collect within nondependent areas. Volumes as small as 1 to 2 cm^3 of air have been reported using this method [8,9]. The instillation of intraluminal water-soluble contrast media in cases of suspected perforation can also improve sensitivity [10].

CT is a widely available imaging tool that is very sensitive for many causes of abdominal pain. With newer rapid helical scanning methods, advances in intravenous and oral contrast agents, three-dimensional reformatting, and other advanced software capabilities, CT has become the imaging modality of choice for the evaluation of most presentations of acute abdominal pain. For example, CT can diagnose acute appendicitis with a reported sensitivity and specificity as high as 98% and 97%, respectively [11]. In fact, the superior diagnostic capability of CT is rendering plain films obsolete. Even in situations in which plain films have a proven diagnostic accuracy, such as perforated viscus or small bowel obstruction, many physicians now opt for CT as the initial imaging study. CT has proven to be more sensitive and specific for nearly all causes of acute abdominal pain [12–14].

Ultrasonography should be the initial imaging modality for patients who are suspected of having biliary tract disease. It is accurate for the detection of gallstones and dilation of the biliary tree. Ultrasonography is less sensitive for choledocholithiasis, and patients who are suspected of having common bile duct stones should be evaluated further with magnetic resonance cholangiopancreatography, endoscopic retrograde cholangiopancreatography (ERCP), or possibly endoscopic ultrasonography. Although MRI can be highly accurate in the diagnosis of acute abdominal pain, its high cost and lack of immediate availability limit its use in the acute care setting.

After clinically evaluating patients who have abdominal pain, the primary physician must appropriately triage the patient. There are several history, physical examination, laboratory, and radiographic red flags that should alert the physician of a potentially more serious cause of the abdominal pain (Box 2). The chronicity of symptoms is an important factor in this decision. Patients with chronic symptoms can usually be evaluated on an outpatient basis. On the other hand, patients who have new-onset symptoms are more likely to have a significant disease process, which can bring harm to them within hours to days. Depending on the differential diagnosis, the physician should consider expediting the evaluation. Although a detailed discussion of all the potential causes of acute abdominal pain is beyond the scope and aim of this article, there are some causes that merit a more detailed discussion. Following is an overview of those causes of abdominal pain that are seen commonly in the outpatient setting, with a focus on causes that are prone to more serious or life-threatening complications. The consideration of most of the following entities should prompt urgent or emergent transfer to an ED or admission to an inpatient hospital bed.

Cholecystitis

Acute cholecystitis is caused most commonly by the obstruction of the cystic duct by a gallstone. More than 90% of cases of cholecystitis are

---

Box 2. Red flags in abdominal pain

History
- Inability to maintain po intake
- Projectile vomiting
- Overt gastrointestinal blood loss
- Syncope
- Pregnancy
- Recent surgery or endoscopic procedure
- Fever
- Caustic or foreign body ingestion

Physical examination
- Pathologic changes in vital signs
- Bloody, maroon, or melenic stool
- Hernia (incarcerated and tender)
- Hypoxia
- Cyanosis
- Altered mentation
- Jaundice
- Peritoneal signs
- Abdominal pain out of proportion to examination

Laboratory results
- Renal failure
- Metabolic acidosis
- Leukocytosis
- Elevated transaminases
- Elevated alkaline phosphatase and bilirubin
- Anemia or polycythemia
- Hyperlipasemia/hyperamylasemia
- Hyperglycemia/hypoglycemia

Radiography
- Abdominal free air
- Gallbladder wall thickening
- Pericholecystic fluid
- Dilated biliary tree
- Bowel obstruction
- Dilated small bowel loops ± air fluid levels
- Intra-abdominal abscess
- Bowel wall thickening
- Air in the portal venous system
- Pneumatosis intestinalis

---

caused by gallstones (calculous cholecystitis) [15]. Simple biliary colic is also caused by gallbladder calculi obstructing the cystic duct, but the duration of obstruction is more short-lived. Generally, biliary colic should not last more than 6 hours, whereas the symptoms of acute cholecystitis last much longer. Prolonged obstruction of the cystic duct impairs gallbladder emptying, leading to inflammation of the gallbladder mucosa. Secondary bacterial infection of the gallbladder may ensue, leading to possible empyema, gallbladder necrosis, and perforation. Approximately 8% to 12% of cases of acute cholecystitis result in gallbladder perforation, carrying a mortality of 20% [9]. Emphysematous cholecystitis, characterized by air in the wall of the gallbladder, is most often seen in patients who have diabetes mellitus.

Approximately 75% of patients who develop acute cholecystitis have a history of biliary colic [16]. The pain caused by biliary colic is a visceral pain that results from tonic spasm of the cystic duct [17]. It is most commonly felt in the epigastrum and may radiate to the right shoulder. The pain has a sudden onset, worsens in severity during the first 15 to 30 minutes, reaches a plateau, and then slowly resolves over the next 6 hours. The pain may be precipitated by fatty food intake, which stimulates gallbladder contraction through the release of cholecystokinin. It is associated commonly with nausea and vomiting. If the pain lasts longer than 6 hours, acute cholecystitis should be suspected. As acute gallbladder inflammation irritates the parietal peritoneum, the pain may shift from the epigastrum to the right upper quadrant.

The physical examination of patients who have acute calculous cholecystitis reveals right upper quadrant tenderness. An inspiratory arrest during deep right upper quadrant palpation is referred to as Murphy's sign.

Frequently encountered laboratory abnormalities include leukocytosis with a left shift and elevation of alkaline phosphatase and transaminase. Generally, hyperbilirubinemia does not occur with acute cholecystitis because the flow of bile through the common bile duct is not impaired. Mirizzi's syndrome is an exception to this rule. Mirizzi's syndrome occurs when a large stone in the cystic duct compresses or erodes into the common hepatic duct, resulting in variable degrees of biliary obstruction.

Right upper quadrant ultrasonography should be the initial imaging test for patients who are suspected of having acute cholecystitis, with reported sensitivity, specificity, and accuracy approaching 95% [9]. Common findings include cholelithiasis, gallbladder wall thickening, pericholecystic fluid, and a sonographic Murphy's sign. The latter finding occurs when the ultrasound transducer pressure on the gallbladder results in tenderness with inspiratory arrest. The finding of cholelithiasis and a positive sonographic Murphy's sign has a positive predictive value (PPV) of 92% for acute cholecystitis. Conversely, when these findings are absent, the negative predictive value (NPV) is 95% [9]. Radionuclide cholescintigraphy scans, such as the hepatobiliary iminodiacetic acid scan, can be used to confirm the diagnosis of acute cholecystitis when ultrasonography findings are equivocal. The sensitivity, specificity, and PPV for acute calculous cholecystitis are 95%, 99%, and 97%, respectively [18].

Acalculous cholecystitis accounts for 5% to 10% of cases of acute cholecystitis [15]. Bile stasis, superconcentration of bile, and gallbladder ischemia are believed to play a role in the pathogenesis. Acalculous cholecystitis is rarely seen in the outpatient setting because it typically occurs in critically ill patients. Furthermore, it tends to carry a higher mortality and perforation rate than calculous cholecystitis, secondary in large part to the severity of comorbid illnesses. Other risk factors include total parenteral nutrition (TPN), diabetes, HIV, prolonged fasting, vasculitides, acute renal failure, and immunosuppression. Idiopathic cases have also been described.

The initial management for acute calculous cholecystitis includes bowel rest, intravenous fluids, analgesia, and parenterally administered antibiotics that cover typical enteric pathogens. The appropriate timing for cholecystectomy has been a much-debated topic, in which most authors favor early surgical intervention. A cholecystectomy performed within 24 to 48 hours of presentation has been shown to reduce mortality and shorten hospital stay compared with surgery performed after weeks of conservative management aimed at "cooling off" the gallbladder [19–21]. The benefits of early cholecystectomy have been validated prospectively for the laparoscopic approach as well [22–26]. The surgical management of acute acalculous cholecystitis is similar to that of calculous cholecystitis but more dependent on the patient's ability to undergo surgery. Many patients who are too ill to undergo surgery are managed acutely with cholecystectomy catheter drainage. Open cholecystectomy has been the traditional approach, but studies have shown that a laparoscopic approach is a safe alternative [27,28].

Cholangitis

Ascending cholangitis is a potentially lethal entity that occurs when the bile ducts become obstructed. Once bile flow is impeded, superinfection of the stagnant bile occurs. Pus builds up under pressure, which causes the infection to rapidly ascend into the liver and spread into the blood stream. Common pathogens include *Escherichia coli*, *Klebsiella* spp, *Bacteroides*, *Enterococcus*, and other enteric pathogens [29]. The most common cause of obstruction in the United States is choledocholithiasis, which accounts for approximately 85% of cases. Although the majority of cases resulting from choledocholithiasis are from gallbladder stones, the in situ formation of common duct stones (primary common bile duct stones) also may occur [30]. Benign biliary strictures, choledochal cysts, biliary parasites, and neoplasms are less common causes of cholangitis.

Symptoms and signs of cholangitis include fever, jaundice, and right upper quadrant pain. These findings are collectively referred to as Charcot's triad, which has a reported sensitivity for cholangitis as high as 75% [31]. As cholangitis progresses, mental obtundation and signs and symptoms of septicemia occur. The combination of Charcot's triad with these findings is known as Reynolds' pentad. Although the sensitivity of Reynolds' pentad is significantly lower than that of Charcot's triad, its presence is significant because it indicates a higher morbidity and mortality rate [15].

Laboratory findings of ascending cholangitis include leukocytosis with a left shift, elevated alkaline phosphatase, and elevation of transaminases. An elevation of pancreatic enzymes can be seen in approximately one third of patients, especially with concomitant gallstone pancreatitis [32]. Because the pathophysiology of this disorder involves common bile duct obstruction, conjugated hyperbilirubinemia is invariably present.

The diagnosis of cholangitis is often made clinically and should be confirmed with cholangiography. Although ultrasonography may suggest the presence of biliary obstruction, its sensitivity for choledocholithiasis is poor [9]. Therefore, when the clinical diagnosis of ascending cholangitis is suspected, patients should undergo cholangiography even in the setting of an unremarkable right upper quadrant ultrasonography.

Patients who are suspected of having acute cholangitis should be referred quickly to an emergency department or hospitalized because the clinical course can progress rapidly and be fatal if left untreated. The initial management should include intravenous fluid resuscitation, bowel rest, and the initiation of broad-spectrum antibiotics with adequate coverage against common enteric pathogens. Patients who are suspected of having cholangitis should have blood drawn and cultured at presentation so that therapy can be directed toward the offending pathogen. Additionally, vitamin K should be administered to patients who have elevated prothrombin time because prolonged biliary obstruction can lead to vitamin K deficiency.

The definitive therapy for cholangitis is decompression of the obstructed biliary system. ERCP is the diagnostic and therapeutic procedure of choice and is successful in relieving the obstruction in more than 95% of cases [18]. This is typically accomplished by stone extraction or the placement of a plastic stent into the common bile duct. In cases in which therapeutic ERCP is not available or is unsuccessful, options include percutaneous transhepatic cholangiography or surgical decompression. If choledocholithiasis is the cause of ascending cholangitis, patients should undergo elective cholecystectomy once the infection resolves.

Pancreatitis

Acute pancreatitis is an inflammatory disease of the pancreas that may cause significant morbidity and carries a case fatality rate of 5% to 9% [33]. Gallstones and alcohol account for more than 80% of cases in the United States [18]. Other less common causes of pancreatitis include medications, trauma, hypercalcemia, severe hypertriglyceridemia (≥ 1000 mg/dL), malignancy, sphincter of Oddi dysfunction, infections, iatrogenic causes (ERCP), and congenital abnormalities of the pancreas such as pancreas divisum. In some cases, the cause of pancreatitis is not determined and is termed idiopathic. As much as 75% of cases of idiopathic pancreatitis are actually caused by biliary sludge or microlithiasis [34]. Regardless of the cause, diffuse pancreatic inflammation and edema develop. In severe cases, necrosis of pancreatic and peripancreatic tissue occurs, and multiorgan failure may ensue. Necrotizing pancreatitis occurs in 25% of patients who have pancreatitis and has a mortality rate of 15% to 20% [33,35].

Patients with pancreatitis present typically with the acute onset of abdominal pain, nausea, and vomiting. The pain is steady and is usually located in the epigastrum, but it may also be appreciated in the right or left upper quadrants of the abdomen. Pain is often described as a boring sensation that radiates into the back. Patients are often unable to get comfortable when lying supinely, and they will lean forward in an attempt to find relief. Because of marked fluid shifts, intravascular volume may become markedly depleted. As a result, tachycardia and hypotension with orthostatic changes may develop. Other vital sign abnormalities include low-grade fever and tachypnea. The latter is a poor prognostic sign and may herald the development of acute respiratory distress syndrome. The abdominal examination may reveal diminished or absent bowel sounds secondary to the development of a paralytic ileus. Abdominal distension may also occur. With palpation, the abdomen may be diffusely tender, but focal tenderness in the epigastrum is more common. Depending on the severity of the pancreatitis, voluntary guarding and rebound tenderness may also be appreciated. Signs of hemorrhagic pancreatitis such as Gray-Turner's sign (flank ecchymosis), Cullen's sign (periumbilical ecchymosis), or Fox's sign (inguinal ecchymosis) are seen in less than 1% of cases. Other rare physical findings of acute pancreatitis include subcutaneous nodules and synovitis, which result from subcutaneous fat necrosis. When acute pancreatitis is suspected clinically, levels of serum amylase or lipase should be determined. In the setting of suspected acute pancreatitis, levels greater than three times the normal values have a high specificity for acute pancreatitis. Serum lipase remains elevated for a longer duration than serum amylase and is more specific for acute pancreatitis [36]. The magnitude of elevation of the serum amylase and lipase does not correlate well with disease severity. As a result of the marked intravascular volume depletion that occurs, the hematocrit is often elevated in acute pancreatitis secondary to hemoconcentration. Hematocrit levels higher than 44% are associated with a worse prognosis [37]. An elevation of ALT to greater than 150 mg/dL suggests gallstones as the cause of the pancreatitis [38]. Hyperbilirubinemia and elevations of the alkaline phosphatase also point to a biliary cause. A bilirubin level greater than 5 mg/dL that does not fall after 6 to 12 hours suggests the presence of an impacted stone in the ampulla of Vater. Because of marked fluid shifts that occur with acute pancreatitis, blood-urea-nitrogen, creatinine, and serum electrolyte levels, including calcium, should be assessed.

Imaging of the pancreas with CT can confirm the diagnosis of acute pancreatitis but is not necessary in all cases. The present authors believe that CT scanning should be reserved for patients in whom the diagnosis is in question, cases of suspected pancreatic necrosis, or in cases of clinical deterioration despite adequate medical therapy. The use of intravenous contrast is highly recommended, and CT should ideally be deferred until the patient has received adequate volume resuscitation to prevent nephrotoxicity.

The care of patients who have acute pancreatitis is complicated by the difficulty in determining whether a patient's course will be mild or severe. Several scoring systems have been developed to assess the severity in acute pancreatitis and to determine prognosis. The most well known of all these criteria is Ranson's criterion, which was originally developed for alcoholic pancreatitis and later modified and validated for gallstone pancreatitis. Ranson's criterion has limited clinical value because it takes 48 hours to determine. The Imrie-Glasgow criteria and the acute physiology and chronic health evaluation II score are two other prospective systems, but both are cumbersome to perform. A prognostic CT scoring system, known as the Balthazar criteria, has been validated for predicting severity in acute pancreatitis. The score is weighted heavily on the presence of pancreatic necrosis [39]. A CT scan can also be used when the diagnosis is in question, but is not necessary in all cases of acute pancreatitis. Specifically, the role of an abdominal CT without intravenous contrast in a dehydrated patient at presentation is miniscule. These authors believe that CT scanning should be reserved for patients in whom the diagnosis is in question, cases of suspected pancreatic necrosis, or in cases of clinical deterioration despite adequate medical therapy. Intravenous contrast is mandatory, and CT should ideally be deferred until the patient has received adequate volume resuscitation.

The cornerstone of therapy in acute pancreatitis is the prevention of pancreatic stimulation. Patients should take nothing orally (NPO) and therefore require a hospital setting for treatment. Both solid food and liquids can stimulate pancreatic secretion; thus, a clear liquid diet is not appropriate until the pain resolves. Aggressive intravenous fluid repletion is necessary to maintain intravascular volume and allow adequate perfusion of the pancreas and extrapancreatic organs such as the kidneys. Other supportive measures include adequate analgesia and the use of nasogastric tubes in patients who experience vomiting secondary to an ileus. Although a clear decline in mortality rate has not been demonstrated with prophylactic antibiotics, the present authors believe that antibiotics should be administered to patients who have necrotizing pancreatitis because they decrease the incidence of septic complications [40]. In patients who are unlikely to resume oral feeding within a few days, enteral nutrition through a nasojejunal tube is preferable to TPN [41–43]. In most cases, supportive care is all that is needed because nearly 90% of patients who have acute pancreatitis will respond to medical management [18]. Patients with gallstone pancreatitis and evidence of ongoing biliary obstruction should undergo ERCP and biliary decompression [44–46].

Appendicitis

Appendicitis is the most common abdominal surgical emergency in the United States, with over 250,000 appendectomies performed annually [47]. Most cases of appendicitis are believed to result from an obstruction of the appendicular lumen by fecaliths. After obstruction, increased intraluminal pressure causes local ischemia, leading to transluminal inflammation. Secondary bacterial infection occurs, and gangrene and perforation of the appendix may result.

A thorough history and physical examination are all that are required to clinically diagnose appendicitis. As a result of appendicular hypertension and distension, a visceral-type pain is felt initially in the periumbilical region. Patients often describe it as crampy in quality. There is often associated nausea, vomiting, and fever. As the inflammatory process progresses and directly irritates the parietal peritoneum, the quality of the pain becomes sharp and shifts to the right lower quadrant (RLQ). Almost all patients who have appendicitis will lose their appetite; in fact, if a patient is hungry, the clinical diagnosis of appendicitis should be questioned.

Auscultation of the abdomen reveals diminished or absent bowel sounds. Classically, the examination of patients who have appendicitis reveals tenderness to palpation at McBurney's point, anatomically located one third of the way from an imaginary line drawn from the anterior superior iliac spine to the umbilicus. Guarding, rigidity, and rebound tenderness may be present from peritoneal irritation. Rovsing's sign may be present, which is the elicitation of RLQ pain on left lower quadrant palpation. The obturator and iliopsoas signs can be elicited by internal rotation of the right hip and extension of the right hip, respectively. These findings occur as the result of the inflammatory process irritating the respective muscles during movement.

Patients who present with acute abdominal pain migrating from the umbilicus to the right lower quadrant and in whom the right lower quadrant is tender to the examiner's touch should undergo emergent appendectomy. The accuracy of the clinical diagnosis in this situation has been estimated to be nearly 95% [48]. However, the classic presentation of appendicitis described above occurs only in an estimated 66% of patients [49]. Atypical presentations account for the remainder, which result from either anomalous appendiceal anatomy or appear in certain populations of patients who are more prone to atypical presentations of common diseases, such as elderly, immunocompromised, or pregnant patients. For example, a retrocecal appendix that becomes inflamed may produce right flank rather than abdominal pain. Patients older than 55 years of age may present with vague symptoms and more subtle examination findings, which cause a delay in the diagnosis. This delay results in a higher rate of perforation compared with their younger counterparts [49]. Finally, misdiagnosis is more common in premenopausal women owing to a broadened gynecologic differential diagnosis and confusing presentations [50].

Leukocytosis is highly sensitive but not specific for the diagnosis of appendicitis [51]. Pyuria, bacteriuria, or hematuria may be seen in up to 40% of presenting patients, making the differentiation problematic between acute appendicitis and urologic infections [52]. In any woman of childbearing age, pregnancy should be ruled out with a serum or urinary β-human chorionic gonadotropin test.

Classic appendicitis is a clinical diagnosis that does not require imaging for confirmation. However, if the diagnosis is uncertain, especially with atypical presentations, imaging can be useful. Plain radiographs are neither sensitive nor specific for the diagnosis of acute appendicitis and should not be ordered [48]. In direct comparison studies, CT has been shown to have a greater sensitivity, accuracy, and negative predictive value than ultrasonography for the diagnosis of acute appendicitis. Ultrasonography has a sensitivity of 75% to 90%, a specificity of 86% to 100%, a PPV of 89% to 93%, and an overall accuracy rate for acute appendicitis of 90% to 94% [53–57]. CT has a sensitivity of 90% to 100%, a specificity of 91% to 99%, a PPV of 95% to 97%, and an overall accuracy rate of 90% to 98% [54,58,59].

Furthermore, compared with ultrasonography, CT is superior in the accurate detection of not only appendicitis but alternative and concomitant abdominal pathology as well [60–62].

Patients with suspected appendicitis should be NPO and started on intravenous fluids. The prophylactic use of antibiotics is not supported by the literature and should be used only in cases of suspected perforation. Because of the potential perforation risk, patients who have a clinical diagnosis of appendicitis should undergo emergent surgical intervention. Historically, a 20% presurgical false-positive rate has been considered acceptable. In patients in whom the clinical diagnosis is uncertain, imaging studies and observation admissions for serial abdominal examinations may decrease this false-positive rate.

Ischemic bowel disease

Depending on the location, degree, and acuity of the vascular compromise, ischemic bowel disease is classified into three distinct syndromes: acute mesenteric ischemia, chronic mesenteric ischemia, and colonic ischemia. Acute mesenteric ischemia results from the rapid loss of blood supply to the portion of the intestines supplied by the celiac, superior mesenteric, or inferior mesenteric arteries. The cause is most commonly thromboembolic disease. The consequences of acute mesenteric ischemia are severe and include bowel necrosis, infarction, and death. Chronic mesenteric ischemia results from the gradual loss of blood supply to the portion of the intestines supplied by the celiac, superior mesenteric, or inferior mesenteric arteries. The cause is usually atherosclerosis. Patients with chronic mesenteric ischemia present with chronic postprandial abdominal pain, called intestinal angina. Because the pain is worsened by eating, patients develop sitophobia (fear of eating), and significant weight loss may occur. Colonic ischemia, also known as ischemic colitis, is the most commonly encountered intestinal vascular disorder [63]. Colonic ischemia occurs when there is a decrease in colonic mucosal oxygenation. In the vast majority of patients, colonic ischemia does not result from an occlusive vascular process, but rather occurs when the oxygen requirements to a specific portion of the colon are not met by the vascular supply. Colonic ischemia occurs in the portions of the colon where blood flow is least redundant, the watershed areas between the superior and inferior mesenteric artery supply, the splenic flexure, and rectosigmoid junction. Lower gastrointestinal bleeding, rather than abdominal pain, is the most common presenting symptom. The disorder is self-limited in most cases, and the prognosis is good. Of the three ischemic bowel syndromes, acute mesenteric ischemia is the disease that presents with acute abdominal pain and will be discussed further below.

The acute interruption of blood supply in the mesenteric vasculature results from either thromboembolic disease or vasospasm. The major risk factors include older age, hypercoagulability, vascular disease, and heart disorders such as atrial fibrillation or valvular disease. Once the blood supply to the mesenteric vascular is interrupted, acute ischemia ensues. If the vascular compromise persists, bowel infarction, necrosis, and perforation may occur. Patients with acute mesenteric ischemia present with an acute onset of severe periumbilical abdominal pain. Early in the disease course, the pain is often out of proportion to the tenderness produced during the physical examination. If the patient presents after bowel infarction has already occurred, peritoneal signs may develop. The stool may be positive for occult blood, but hematochezia is uncommon with acute mesenteric ischemia.

Common laboratory test abnormalities seen with acute mesenteric ischemia include leukocytosis and an elevated hematocrit from hemoconcentration. A low level of serum bicarbonate, metabolic acidosis, and an elevated lactate level are seen once bowel infarction has already occurred. Retrospective studies evaluating the role of elevated plasma D-dimer levels in the diagnosis of early mesenteric ischemia have shown initial promise, although subsequent prospective evaluations have shown D-dimer to be less helpful [64,65].

Several imaging modalities, including plain films, Doppler ultrasonography, conventional CT, and MRI have been studied for the diagnosis of acute mesenteric ischemia. Unfortunately, these imaging techniques lack sensitivity and specificity for an accurate diagnosis [66]. Mesenteric angiography is the gold standard test for diagnosing occlusive arterial mesenteric ischemia. Its sensitivity and specificity are 75% to 100% and 100%, respectively [63]. In addition to its diagnostic capabilities, angiography offers the potential for treatment. Several studies demonstrate a decreased mortality in patients who undergo routine angiography for suspected occlusive mesenteric arterial ischemia [67,68].

The mortality rate for patients who have acute mesenteric ischemia that has not been diagnosed before the onset of bowel infarction is reportedly as high as 90% [63]; therefore, early diagnosis is crucial. Because laboratory findings may be nonspecific early in the disease course, a high index of suspicion based on predisposing risk factors and clinical presentation are required. Patients presenting with suspected acute mesenteric ischemia should promptly undergo angiography and surgical evaluation [69].

Diverticulitis

Diverticular disease of the colon is common and increases with age. Nearly one third of patients over the age of 50 and two thirds by the age of 80 have diverticular disease [70]. Diverticulitis, a complication caused by the perforation of a diverticulum, affects up to 25% of patients who have diverticular disease [71]. Inspissated food, stool, and increased intraluminal pressure are believed to be involved in the pathogenesis of diverticular perforation. The clinical presentation of patients who have diverticulitis depends on the extent of the perforation. Small perforations are walled off by surrounding mesentery and pericolonic fat, whereas larger perforations can result in extensive intraperitoneal abscess formation and frank peritonitis.

The location of abdominal pain in patients who have diverticulitis depends on the location of the perforated diverticulum. Because diverticular disease most commonly affects the sigmoid colon, patients most often present with crampy left lower quadrant abdominal pain. However, right lower quadrant abdominal pain may occur in patients who have a redundant sigmoid colon or diverticular disease involving the right colon [72]. Nausea, vomiting, fever, and anorexia are associated symptoms. Physical examination often reveals tenderness over the inflamed area, and an inflammatory mass may be palpable. In patients who have free perforation, diffuse peritoneal signs such as rebound, guarding, and rigidity may be present.

Although diverticulitis often can be diagnosed on clinical grounds alone, an imaging study should be performed during a patient's initial presentation to confirm the presence of the diverticulae. A CT of the abdomen and pelvis with intravenous, oral, and optional rectal contrast is the diagnostic modality of choice, with a reported sensitivity as high as 98% [73]. Colonoscopy should not be performed in patients who are suspected of having diverticulitis because perforation is a contraindication for the procedure.

Mild, uncomplicated diverticulitis can be managed on an outpatient basis and consists of a clear liquid diet and the administration of oral antibiotics that cover typical gastrointestinal pathogens. Complicated diverticulitis occurs when patients develop intra-abdominal abscesses, fistulas, free perforations, or intestinal obstructions and require hospitalization. Enteral feedings should be held, and patients are started on intravenous antibiotics. Intra-abdominal abscesses can often be managed with percutaneous drainage catheters, but surgery is sometimes required [74]. Free perforation or intestinal obstruction usually mandates emergent surgery.

Obstruction

Bowel obstruction occurs when the normal flow of intestinal contents is interrupted by a mechanical blockage. Approximately 75% of cases of small bowel obstruction (SBO) is the result of adhesive peritoneal bands in patients who have a history of abdominal surgery [75,76]. In fact, up to 15% of patients who undergo laparotomy will be readmitted within 2 years with SBO from adhesions, and up to 3% will require operative intervention as a result [77]. Furthermore, it is estimated that the 10-year risk of developing recurrent SBO from adhesions is approximately 40% [78]. Hernias are the second most common cause of SBO and account for up to 25% of cases [79]. The remaining cases of SBO result from a number of causes, including Crohn's disease, volvulus, neoplasm, intussusception, gallstones, and ischemia.

Once the bowel is obstructed, the segment of bowel proximal to the obstruction becomes increasingly distended by swallowed air, gas from bacterial fermentation, and luminal secretions. Bacterial overgrowth, bowel edema, and the loss of absorptive function follow. If the obstruction is not treated promptly, ischemia, necrosis, and perforation may occur.

The pain caused by small bowel obstruction is a colicky, diffuse pain, which waxes and wanes over 5-minute intervals. Nausea, vomiting, distention, and obstipation are associated with the pain. The emesis is often feculent because of bacterial overgrowth. The passage of stool and flatus do not eliminate SBO from the differential diagnosis because luminal contents distal to the blockage can still pass. Physical examination reveals a distended, diffusely tender abdomen with either hyperactive high-pitched or hypoactive bowel sounds. Rushes of luminal fluid can often be heard. Findings of rigidity, rebound tenderness, or guarding suggest peritonitis. A ventral, inguinal, or periumbilical hernia should be sought as a potential cause. Patients will often exhibit physical signs of dehydration. Laboratory analysis is usually nonspecific, but common abnormalities include hemoconcentration, leukocytosis, and electrolyte imbalances.

An abdominal plain film series should be the initial diagnostic imaging test in patients who are suspected of having obstruction. Typical findings include air-fluid levels, small bowel distention, and a paucity of air in the rectal vault. In addition, evidence of complications such as intraperitoneal free air can be seen. Although most cases can be diagnosed clinically, with the comfirmatory assistance of plain films, there are instances in which plain films are not sufficient. In these instances, CT may be helpful for both diagnosing SBO and determining the cause, with a reported sensitivity of 100% and accuracy of 90% [80,81].

The clinical presentation of large bowel obstruction (LBO) is very similar to that of SBO. Nearly 60% of cases of LBO are the result of malignancy, with colon cancer being the most common. Other causes include diverticular strictures and colonic volvulus [82]. The cecum and the sigmoid colon are the most common locations of colonic volvulus [83].

Patients with bowel obstructions are initially managed with strict restriction of oral intake, nasogastric tube decompression, intravenous fluids, and electrolyte repletion. Early surgical evaluation is mandatory. The philosophy that "the sun should never rise nor set on a small bowel obstruction" remains true today.

Peptic ulcer disease

Peptic ulcer disease (PUD) is a common condition that has a significant impact on quality of life. In 1989, more than $5 billion was spent on the care of patients who had PUD [84]. The most common cause of PUD is infection by *Helicobacter pylori*. *H pylori* infection has been associated with 75% to 95% of duodenal ulcers and 65% to 95% of gastric ulcers [85–87].

Nonsteroidal anti-inflammatory medications (NSAIDs) are the second most common cause of PUD, with an estimated yearly incidence of clinically significant gastric or duodenal ulceration of approximately 1.5% [88]. The use of NSAIDs presents a particular challenge because up to 40% of patients will not report the use of NSAIDs [89]. Acid hypersecretory syndromes such as Zollinger-Ellison syndrome account for the majority of the remaining cases.

The clinical presentation of PUD depends on the location of the ulcer and whether complications develop from the ulcer. Patients who have uncomplicated peptic ulcers may be asymptomatic or they may present with upper abdominal pain [90,91]. The pain is typically described as a burning or gnawing pain but may occasionally be crampy in nature. Nausea and vomiting may also be seen. In patients who have gastric ulcers, the pain is often made worse by eating, whereas patients who have duodenal ulcers often feel better with eating.

Complications of PUD include bleeding, obstruction, perforation and penetration into adjacent structures. Bleeding from PUD may present with melena, hematochezia, and hematemesis with or without hemodynamic compromise. Bleeding can generally be managed medically with IV fluid, blood transfusions, antisecretory therapy, and endoscopic therapy. Endoscopy is also useful to determine the risk for recurrent bleeding [92]. Surgical or angiographic intervention is reserved for bleeding refractory to endoscopic therapies. Pyloric channel and duodenal bulb ulcers may cause gastric outlet obstruction. In addition to epigastric pain, patients may present nausea, projectile vomiting, early satiety, anorexia and weight loss. Conservative measures are often successful in resolution, though many patients will require surgery or endoscopic dilatation therapy [93,94]. Most ulcers that perforate are located in the duodenal bulb, and are often associated with NSAID use [95,96]. Patients present with the sudden onset of epigastric pain which quickly becomes diffuse as generalized peritonitis ensues. Patients can sometimes develop paradoxical improvement in their pain following perforation despite a markedly rigid and diffusely tender abdomen. Plain films are usually adequate to confirm the diagnosis of ulcer perforation. Perforations require immediate surgical evaluation. Ulcer penetration into adjacent structures occurs in up to 20% of cases of PUD, but only a small proportion become clinically apparent [97]. The most common sites of ulcer penetration include the pancreas, omentum, hepatobiliary system, colon, and adjacent vasculature. Patient presentation reflects the structure that is involved, and the therapy is site-specific.

Summary

Because there are many causes of acute abdominal pain, a systematic approach by the evaluating physician is necessary to narrow the differential diagnosis. It is vital that the physician have an understanding of the mechanisms of pain generation and be familiar with the presentations of common diseases that cause abdominal pain. Recognizing the red flags in the history and physical examination and the initial imaging and laboratory findings helps to determine which patients may have a serious underlying disease process, and therefore warrant more expedited evaluation and treatment.

References

[1] McCraig L, Burt CW. National ambulatory medical care survey: 2002 emergency department summary. Advance Data 2004;340.
[2] Woodnell DA, Cherry DK. National ambulatory medical care survey. 2002 Advance Data 2004;346.
[3] Glasgow RE, Mulvihill SJ. Abdominal pain. In: Feldman M, Friedman LS, Sleisenger MH, editors. Sleisenger and Fordtran's gastrointestinal and liver disease: pathophysiology, diagnosis, management. 7th edition. Philadelphia: WB Saunders; 2002. p. 71–82.
[4] Benedict M, Bucheli B, Battegay E, et al. First clinical judgment by primary care physicians distinguishes well between organic and nonorganic causes of abdominal or chest pain. J Gen Intern Med 1997;12(8):459–65.
[5] Yamamoto W, Kono H, Maekawa M, et al. The relationship between abdominal pain regions and specific diseases: an epidemiologic approach to clinical practice. J Epidemiol 1997;7(1):27–32.
[6] Manimaran N, Galland RB. Significance of routine digital rectal examination in adults presenting with abdominal pain. Ann R Coll Surg Engl 2004;86(4):292–5.
[7] Maglinte DDT, Balthazar EJ, Kelvin FM, et al. The role of radiography in the diagnosis of small bowel obstruction. AJR Am J Roentgenol 1997;168(5):1171–80.
[8] Miller RE, Nelson SW. The roentographic demonstration of tiny amounts of free intraperitoneal gas: experimental and clinical studies. AJR Am J Roentgenol 1971;112(3): 574–85.
[9] Billittier AJ, Abrams BJ, Brunetto A. Radiographic imaging modalities for the patient in the emergency department with abdominal complaints. Emerg Med Clin North Am 1996;14(4): 789–850.
[10] Roh JJ, Thompson JS, Harned RK, et al. Value of pneumoperitoneum in the diagnosis of visceral perforation. Am J Surg 1983;146(6):830–3.
[11] Gupta H, Dupuy D. Advances in imaging of the acute abdomen. Surg Clin North Am 1997; 77(6):1245–63.
[12] Ahn SH, Mayo-Smith WW, Murphy BL, et al. Acute nontraumatic abdominal pain in adult patients: abdominal radiography compared with CT evaluation. Radiology 2002;225(1): 159–64.
[13] Tsushima Y, Yamada S, Aoki J, et al. Effect of contrast-enhanced computed tomography on diagnosis and management of acute abdomen in adults. Clin Radiol 2002;57(6):507–13.
[14] Stapakis JP, Thickman D. Diagnosis of pneumoperitoneum: abdominal CT vs. upright chest film. J Comput Assist Tomogr 1992;16(5):713–6.
[15] Yusoff IF, Barkun JS, Barkun AN. Diagnosis and management of cholecystitis and cholangitis. Gastroenterol Clin North Am 2003;32(4):1145–68.
[16] Raine PA, Gunn AA. Acute cholecystitis. Br J Surg 1975;62(9):697–700.
[17] Sullivan FJ, Eaton SB Jr, Ferrucci JT Jr, et al. Cholangiographic manifestations of acute biliary colic. N Engl J Med 1973;288(1):33–5.
[18] Kadakia SC. Biliary tract emergencies. Med Clin North Am 1993;77(5):1015–36.
[19] van der Linden W, Sunzel H. Early versus delayed operation for acute cholecystitis: a controlled trial. Am J Surg 1970;120(1):7–13.

[20] McArthur P, Cuschieri A, Sells R, et al. Controlled clinical trial comparing early with interval cholecystectomy for acute cholecystitis. Br J Surg 1975;62(10):850–2.

[21] Jarvinen H, Hastbacka J. Early cholecystectomy for acute cholecystitis: a prospective randomized trial. Ann Surg 1980;191(4):501–5.

[22] Lai PB, Kwong KH, Leung KL, et al. Randomized trial of early versus late laparoscopic cholecystectomy for acute cholecystitis. Br J Surg 1998;85(6):764–7.

[23] Lo CM, Liu CL, Fan ST, et al. Prospective randomized study of early versus late laparoscopic cholecystectomy for acute cholecystitis. Ann Surg 1998;227(4):461–7.

[24] Chandler CF, Lane JS, Ferguson P, et al. Prospective evaluation of early versus delayed laparoscopic cholecystectomy for treatment of acute cholecystitis. Am Surg 2000;66(9):896–900.

[25] Brodsky A, Matter I, Sabo E, et al. Laparoscopic cholecystectomy for acute cholecystitis: can the need for conversion and the probability for complications be predicted? Surg Endosc 2000;14(8):755–60.

[26] Pessaux P, Teuch JJ, Rouge C, et al. Laparoscopic cholecystectomy in acute cholecystitis: a prospective comparative study in patients with acute vs. chronic cholecystitis. Surg Endosc 2000;14(4):358–61.

[27] Lillemoe KD. Surgical treatment of biliary tract infections. Am Surg 2000;66(2):138–44.

[28] Kalliafas S, Ziegler DW, Flancbaum L, et al. Acute acalculous cholecystitis: incidence, risk factors, diagnosis, and outcome. Am Surg 1998;64(5):471–5.

[29] Maluenda F, Csendes A, Burdiles P, et al. Bacteriologic study of choledocal bile in patients with common bile duct stones, with or without acute suppurative cholangitis. Hepatogastroenterology 1989;36(3):132–5.

[30] Saharia PC, Zuidema GD, Cameron JL. Primary common duct stones. Ann Surg 1977;185(5):598–604.

[31] Saik RP, Greenburg AG, Farris JM, et al. Spectrum of cholangitis. Am J Surg 1975;130(2):143–50.

[32] Lipsett PA, Pitt HA. Acute cholangitis. Surg Clin North Am 1990;70(6):1297–312.

[33] Banks PA. Practice guidelines in acute pancreatitis. Am J Gastroenterol 1997;92(3):377–86.

[34] Ros E, Navarro S, Bru C, et al. Occult microlithiasis in "idiopathic" acute pancreatitis: prevention of relapses by cholecystectomy or ursodeoxycholic acid therapy. Gastroenterology 1991;101(6):1701–9.

[35] Gullo L, Migliori M, Olah A, et al. Acute pancreatitis in five European countries: etiology and mortality. Pancreas 2002;24(3):223–7.

[36] Steinberg WM, Goldstein SS, Davis ND, et al. Diagnostic assays in acute pancreatitis: a study of sensitivity and specificity. Ann Intern Med 1985;102(5):576–80.

[37] Brown A, Baillargeon J-D, Hughes MD, et al. Can fluid resuscitation prevent pancreatic necrosis in severe acute pancreatitis? Pancreatology 2002;2(2):104–7.

[38] Tenner S, Dubner H, Steinberg W. Predicting gallstone pancreatitis with laboratory parameters: a meta-analysis. Am J Gastroenterol 1994;89(10):1863–6.

[39] Simchuk EJ, Traverso LW, Nukui Y, et al. Computed tomography severity index is a predictor of outcomes for severe pancreatitis. Am J Surg 2000;179(5):352–5.

[40] Pederzoli P, Bassi C, Vesentini S, et al. A randomized multicenter trial of antibiotic prophylaxis of septic complications in acute necrotizing pancreatitis with imipenem. Surg Gynecol Obstet 1993;176(5):480–3.

[41] Olah A, Pardavi G, Belagyi T, et al. Early nasojejunal feeding in acute pancreatitis is associated with a lower complication rate. Nutrition 2002;18(3):259–62.

[42] Kalferentzos F, Kehagias J, Mead N, et al. Enteral nutrition is superior to parenteral nutrition in severe acute pancreatitis: results of a randomized prospective trial. Br J Surg 1997;84(12):1665–9.

[43] Abou-Assi S, Craid K, O'Keefe SJ. Hypocaloric jejunal feeding is better than total parenteral nutrition in acute pancreatic: results of a randomized comparative study. Am J Gastroenterol 2002;97(10):2255–62.

[44] Tenner S. Initial management of acute pancreatitis: critical issues during the first 72 hours. Am J Gastroenterol 2004;99(12):2489–94.

[45] Neoptolemos JP, Carr-Locke DL, London NJ, et al. Controlled trial of urgent endoscopic retrograde cholangiopancreatography and endoscope sphincterotomy versus conservative management for acute pancreatitis due to gallstones. Lancet 1998;2:979–83.

[46] Fan ST, Lai EC, Mok FP, et al. Early treatment of acute biliary pancreatitis by endoscopic papillotomy. N Engl J Med 1993;328(4):228–32.

[47] Owings MF, Kozak LJ. Ambulatory and inpatient procedures in the United States, 1996. Vital and Health Statistics, series 13. National Health Survey. 1998;139:26.

[48] Paulson EK, Kalady MF, Pappas TN. Suspected appendicitis. N Engl J Med 2003;348(3): 236–42.

[49] Graffeo CS, Counselman FL. Appendicitis. Emerg Med Clin North Am 1996;14(4):653–71.

[50] Rothrock SG, Green SM, Dobson M, et al. Misdiagnosis of appendicitis in nonpregnant women of childbearing age. J Emerg Med 1995;13(1):1–8.

[51] Vermeulen B, Morabia A. Influence of white cell count in surgical decision making. Eur J Surg 1995;161(7):483–6.

[52] Puskar D, Bedalov G, Fridrih S, et al. Urinalysis, ultrasound analysis, and renal dynamic scintigraphy in acute appendicitis. Urology 1995;45(1):108–12.

[53] Jahn H, Mathieson FK, Neckelmann K, et al. Comparison of clinical judgment and diagnostic ultrasonography in the diagnosis of acute appendicitis: experience with a score-aided diagnosis. Eur J Surg 1997;163(6):433–43.

[54] Birnbaum BA, Wilson SR. Appendicitis at the millennium. Radiology 2000;215(2): 337–48.

[55] Birnbaum BA, Jeffrey RB Jr. CT and sonographic evaluation of acute right lower quadrant abdominal pain. AJR Am J Roentgenol 1998;170(2):361–71.

[56] Jeffrey RB Jr, Laing FC, Townsend RR. Acute appendicitis: sonographic criteria based on 250 cases. Radiology 1988;167(2):327–9.

[57] Abu-Yousef MM, Bleicher J, Maher JJ, et al. High-resolution sonography of acute appendicitis. AJR Am J Roentgenol 1987;149(1):53–8.

[58] Lane MJ, Liu DM, Huynh MD, et al. Suspected acute appendicitis: nonenhanced helical CT in 300 consecutive patients. Radiology 1999;213(2):341–6.

[59] Raman SS, Lu DS, Kadell BM, et al. Accuracy of nonfocused helical CT for the diagnosis of acute appendicitis: a 5-year review. AJR Am J Roentgenol 2002;178(6):1319–25.

[60] Balthazar EJ, Birnbaum BA, Yee J, et al. Acute appendicitis: CT and US correlation in 100 patients. Radiology 1994;190(1):31–5.

[61] Pickuth D, Heywang-Kobrunner SH, Spielmann RP. Suspected acute appendicitis: is ultrasonography or computed tomography the preferred imaging technique? Eur J Surg 2000; 166(4):315–9.

[62] Terasawa T, Blackmore CC, Bent S, et al. Systematic review: computed tomography and ultrasonography to detect acute appendicitis in adults and adolescents. Ann Intern Med 2004; 141(7):537–46.

[63] Walker JS, Dire DJ. Vascular abdominal emergencies. Emerg Med Clin North Am 1996; 14(3):571–92.

[64] Acosta S, Nilsson TK, Bjorck M. Preliminary study of D-dimer as a possible marker of acute bowel ischaemia. Br J Surg 2001;88(3):385–8.

[65] Acosta S, Nilsson TK, Bjorck M. D-dimer testing in patients with suspected acute thromboembolic occlusion of the superior mesenteric artery. Br J Surg 2004;91(8):991–4.

[66] Lefkovitz Z, Cappell MS, Lookstein R, et al. Radiologic diagnosis and treatment of gastrointestinal hemorrhage and ischemia. Med Clin North Am 2002;86(6):1357–99.

[67] Boos S. Angiography of the mesenteric artery 1976 to 1991: a change in the indications during mesenteric circulatory disorders. Radiologe 1992;32(4):154–7.

[68] Clark RA, Gallant TE. Acute mesenteric ischemia: angiographic spectrum. Am J Radiol 1984;142(3):555–62.

[69] Kaleya R, Sammartano R, Boley SJ. Aggressive approach to acute mesenteric ischemia. Surg Clin North Am 1992;35(6):613–23.

[70] Freeman SR, McNally PR. Diverticulitis. Med Clin North Am 1993;77(5):1149–67.

[71] Parks TG. Natural history of diverticular disease of the colon. Clinics in Gastroenterology 1975;4:53–69.

[72] Markham NI, Li AK. Diverticulitis of the right colon: experience from Hong Kong. Gut 1992;33(4):547–9.

[73] Ambrosetti P, Jenny A, Becker C, et al. Acute left colonic diverticulitis: compared performance of computed tomography and water-soluble contrast enema: prospective evaluation of 420 patients. Dis Colon Rectum 2000;43(10):1363–7.

[74] Schecter S, Eisenstat TE, Oliver GC, et al. Computerized tomographic scan-guided drainage of intra-abdominal abscesses: preoperative and postoperative modalities in colon and rectal surgery. Dis Colon Rectum 1994;37(10):984–8.

[75] Bizer LS, Liebling RW, Delany HM, et al. Small bowel obstruction: the role of nonoperative treatment in simple intestinal obstruction and predictive criteria for strangulation obstruction. Surgery 1981;89(4):407–13.

[76] Greene WW. Bowel obstruction in the aged patient: a review of 300 cases. Am J Surg 1969; 118(4):541–5.

[77] Beck DE, Opelka FG, Bailey HR, et al. Incidence of small-bowel obstruction and adhesiolysis after open colorectal and general surgery. Dis Colon Rectum 1999;42(2):241–8.

[78] Landercasper J, Cogbill TH, Merry WH, et al. Long-term outcome after hospitalization for small-bowel obstruction. Arch Surg 1993;128(7):765–70.

[79] Mucha P Jr. Small intestinal obstruction. Surg Clin North Am 1987;67(3):597–620.

[80] Frager D. Intestinal obstruction: role of CT. Gastroenterol Clin North Am 2002;31(3):777–99.

[81] Frager D, Baer JW, Medwid SW, et al. Detection of intestinal ischemia in patients with acute small-bowel obstruction due to adhesions or hernia: efficacy of CT. AJR Am J Roentgenol 1996;166(1):67–71.

[82] Kahi CJ, Rex DR. Bowel obstruction and pseudo-obstruction. Gastroenterol Clin North Am 2003;32(4):1229–47.

[83] Ballantyne GH, Brandner MD, Beart RW Jr, et al. Volvulus of the colon: incidence and mortality. Ann Surg 1985;202(1):83–92.

[84] Sonnenberg A, Everhart JE. Health impact of peptic ulcer in the US. Am J Gastroenterol 1997;92(4):614–20.

[85] Borody TJ, George LL, Brandl S, et al. *Helicobacter pylori*-negative duodenal ulcer. Am J Gastroenterol 1991;86(9):1154–7.

[86] Ciociola AA, McSorley DJ, Turner K, et al. *Helicobacter pylori* infection rates in duodenal ulcer patients in the United States may be lower than previously estimated. Am J Gastroenterol 1999;94(7):1834–40.

[87] Tytgat G, Langenberg W, Rauws E, et al. Campylobacter-like organism (CLO) in the human stomach [abstract]. Gastroenterology 1985;88(5):1620.

[88] Silverstein FE, Graham DY, Senior JR, et al. Misoprostol reduces serious gastrointestinal complications in patients with rheumatoid arthritis receiving nonsteroidal anti-inflammatory drugs: a randomized, double-blind, placebo-controlled trial. Ann Intern Med 1995; 123(4):241–9.

[89] Lanas AI, Remacha B, Esteva F, et al. Risk factors associated with refractory peptic ulcers. Gastroenterology 1995;109(4):1124–33.

[90] Kuipers EJ, Thijs JC, Festen HP. The prevalence of *Helicobacter pylori* in peptic ulcer disease. Aliment Pharmacol Ther 1995;9(Suppl 2):S59.

[91] Hilton D, Iman N, Burke GJ, et al. Absence of abdominal pain in older persons with endoscopic ulcers: a prospective study. Am J Gastroenterol 2001;96:380.

[92] Laine L, Cohen H, Brodhead J, et al. Prospective evaluation of immediate versus delayed refeeding and prognostic value of endoscopy in patients with upper gastrointestinal hemorrhage. Gastroenterology 1992;102(2):314–6.

[93] Weiland D, Dunn DH, Humphrey EW, et al. Gastric outlet obstruction in peptic ulcer disease: an indication for surgery. Am J Surg 1982;143(1):90–3.

[94] Boylan JJ, Gradzka MI. Long-term results of endoscopic balloon dilatation for gastric outlet obstruction. Dig Dis Sci 1999;44(9):1833–6.

[95] Gunshefski L, Flancbaum L, Brolin RE, et al. Changing patterns in perforated peptic ulcer disease. Am Surg 1990;56(4):270–4.

[96] Lanas A, Serrano P, Bajador E, Esteva F, et al. Evidence of aspirin use in both upper and lower gastrointestinal perforation. Gastroenterology 1997;112(3):683–9.

[97] Norris JR, Haubrich WS. The incidence and clinical features of penetration in peptic ulceration. JAMA 1961;178:386–9.

THE MEDICAL
CLINICS
OF NORTH AMERICA

ELSEVIER
SAUNDERS

Med Clin N Am 90 (2006) 505–523

Back Pain Emergencies

Michael E. Winters, MD[a,b,c,*], Paul Kluetz, MD[a],
Jeffrey Zilberstein, MD[c]

[a]Department of Medicine, University of Maryland School of Medicine, Baltimore, MD, USA
[b]Division of Emergency Medicine, Department of Surgery, University of Maryland School of
Medicine, Baltimore, MD, USA
[c]Combined Internal Medicine and Emergency Medicine Residency Program,
University of Maryland Medical Center, Baltimore, MD, USA

There is, perhaps, no other chief complaint that creates such an overwhelming sense of despair as back pain. In the United States, it is estimated that up to 90% of adults will experience an episode of back pain during their lifetime [1–5]. Most of these patients will present to an office-based physician for initial evaluation and treatment [6]. Back pain is second only to upper respiratory problems as a symptom-related reason to visit a primary care physician [1,5,7,8]. Of the patients who have acute back pain, 90% to 95% have a non–life-threatening condition [8,9]; although up to 85% cannot be given an exact diagnosis, nearly all recover within 4 to 6 weeks [5,8–10].

In the remaining 5% to 10% of patients, acute back pain is a manifestation of more serious pathology. Vascular catastrophes, malignancy, spinal cord compressive syndromes, and infectious disease processes may all present with acute back pain. Although collectively these conditions account for a small percentage of causes of back pain, all are potentially life threatening and require rapid diagnosis. When the diagnosis is missed or even delayed, patients incur substantially higher morbidity and mortality. Thus, it is imperative that the practicing physician be able to recognize which patients who have acute back pain harbor more serious etiologies.

This article reviews various medical emergencies that can present with the symptom of acute back pain. Following a discussion on identifying key components within the history and physical examination, the remainder of the article is dedicated to a review of specific back pain "emergencies." Armed with this information, the practicing internist can promptly

---

* Corresponding author. 1406 Chessie Court, Mt. Airy, MD 21771.
E-mail address: mwint001@umaryland.edu (M.E. Winters).

0025-7125/06/$ - see front matter © 2006 Elsevier Inc. All rights reserved.
doi:10.1016/j.mcna.2005.11.002
medical.theclinics.com

recognize, diagnose, and treat patients who have potentially life-threatening causes of back pain.

History and physical examination: in search of the red flag

The history and physical examination form the cornerstone of the evaluation of the patient who has back pain. As stated, most patients have non–life-threatening conditions and recover within several weeks. Thus, it is not cost-effective or recommended to pursue an exhaustive diagnostic evaluation on every patient. Rather, diagnostic studies are obtained based on the identification of key clinical findings within the history and physical examination. Referred to as red flags, these findings indicate the possibility of serious pathology. The detection of any red flag warrants further investigation. Given their clinical implications, it is useful to review these concerning signs and symptoms. A summary of the following is provided in Box 1.

Box 1. The red flags of back pain

History
Gradual onset of back pain
Age <20 years or >50 years
Thoracic back pain
Pain lasting longer than 6 weeks
History of trauma
Fever/chills/night sweats
Unintentional weight loss
Pain worse with recumbency
Pain worse at night
Unrelenting pain despite supratherapeutic doses of analgesics
History of malignancy
History of immunosuppression
Recent procedure known to cause bacteremia
History of intravenous drug use

Physical examination
Fever
Hypotension
Extreme hypertension
Pale, ashen appearance
Pulsatile abdominal mass
Pulse amplitude differentials
Spinous process tenderness
Focal neurologic signs
Acute urinary retention

History of present illness

Often, the history provides the most useful information in identifying patients who have potentially serious disease. For a systematic approach to identifying red flags, the authors suggest using the pneumonic OLDCAAR (onset, location, duration, context, associated symptoms, aggravating factors, and relieving factors) (Amal Mattu, MD, personal communication, 2005).

Onset

The gradual onset of back pain is a red flag for serious pathology. Back pain that begins or progresses over a period of weeks to months must raise suspicion for malignancy or infection [11]. It is also crucial to note the patient's age at the onset of pain. Back pain that begins before age 20 years suggests congenital or developmental disorders such as spondylolisthesis or spondylolysis [5,9]. Equally concerning is the onset of back pain in patients older than 50 years. In the older patient, new-onset back pain is more likely to be a manifestation of serious conditions such as an abdominal aortic aneurysm (AAA), malignancy, or compression fracture [12]. A new diagnosis of musculoskeletal strain should be a diagnosis of exclusion in the elderly patient.

Location

Beware the patient who has thoracic back pain. Isolated thoracic back pain is a red flag for a variety of medical emergencies. Aortic dissection (AD), spinal epidural abscess (SEA), vertebral osteomyelitis, malignancy, and perforated gastric ulcer are just some of the emergencies that can present with thoracic back pain [13]. Any patient who has thoracic pain, especially in the absence of lumbar pain, must undergo further evaluation. Because most patients who have lumbar strain report paraspinal discomfort, localization of pain to the midline should also raise concern over more serious pathology. Malignancy, vertebral osteomyelitis, fracture, and SEA more commonly produce midline back pain.

Duration

Nearly all patients who have musculoskeletal etiologies of back pain recover within 4 to 6 weeks [8–10]. Back pain that persists longer than 6 weeks is a red flag for conditions such as malignancy or infection. These etiologies should also be considered in the patient whose pain persists despite appropriate conservative management.

Context

Back pain that begins following major trauma such as a motor vehicle accident must raise suspicion for vertebral fracture. Close attention should be paid to elderly patients, especially those who have osteoporosis. Even minimal trauma in these patients, such as a fall, can result in a vertebral fracture [12]. Patients should be questioned about recent procedures. Back pain that develops in the context of a recent procedure such as those involving the genitourinary or gastrointestinal system is at risk for infectious etiologies. These procedures are known to have a relatively high incidence of bacteremia and can result in hematogenous seeding of the spine [5].

Associated symptoms

Any patient who has back pain must be questioned about the presence of associated neurologic symptoms. Any report of parasthesias, motor weakness, urinary or fecal incontinence, or gait abnormalities mandates additional evaluation. Any patient who has back pain and urinary or fecal abnormalities should be considered to have spinal cord compression until proved otherwise [5]. Equally concerning is the presence of fever, night sweats, malaise, or unintentional weight loss. These associated symptoms indicate the possibility of malignancy or infection.

Aggravating factors

Back pain that is aggravated by lying down is a red flag for malignancy or infection [9]. These etiologies must also be considered in the patient who reports pain that awakens them at night. Pain that is worse at night is atypical for musculoskeletal etiologies and, if present, warrants further investigation.

Relieving factors

Pain that improves with sitting or slight flexion of the spine indicates the diagnosis of spinal stenosis [14]. In addition to body position or maneuvers, patients should also be questioned regarding the effect of analgesic medication. Patients whose pain is unremitting despite supratherapeutic doses of medications must be evaluated for more serious causes of back pain.

Past medical history

Aside from features of the history of present illness, there are components of the past medical history that should raise suspicion for nonmusculoskeletal etiologies of back pain. Patients who have poorly controlled hypertension are at risk for an AD or rupturing AAA. Immunocompromised patients such as those who have HIV, organ transplantation, diabetes, or prolonged steroid use are at greater risk for an infectious etiology. Any patient who has back pain and a previous history of cancer must be evaluated for spinal epidural metastases (SEM). Back pain is often the initial presenting symptom in a number of patients found to have metastatic disease [15].

Social history

All patients must be questioned regarding the use of illicit substances. Any patient who has back pain and uses intravenous drugs must be emergently evaluated for SEA. Similarly, chronic use of tobacco is the strongest independent risk factor for the development of an AAA [16].

Physical examination

Physical examination of the patient who has back pain begins with an assessment of vital signs. Any patient who has back pain, abdominal pain, and hypotension must be considered to have a rupturing AAA until proved otherwise. Conversely, marked hypertension and thoracic back pain should raise concern over AD. The presence of fever is considered by many to be a red flag for infectious pathology [5,17]. Caution must be used when interpreting temperature, however, because the sensitivity of fever ranges from 27% to 83% [17]. The lack of fever is insufficient to rule out an infectious cause of back pain.

Immediate concern must be raised for the patient who appears pale, ashen, or diaphoretic. More often, these patients have life-threatening etiologies such as AD or rupturing AAA. Similar concern should be raised for the patient who is unable to remain still. Nearly all patients who have musculoskeletal strain prefer to remain immobile because any movement exacerbates symptoms. Patients who pace about the examining room should be suspected to have renal colic, pyelonephritis, or in rare cases, spinal infection.

To avoid potentially costly diagnostic delays, examination of related organ systems should be performed before proceeding directly to the back. Meticulous attention to the cardiovascular, pulmonary, gastrointestinal, and urogenital systems is warranted because disease processes in any one of these systems can cause acute back pain. When examining the back, the clinician should note any cutaneous findings that suggest infection or trauma. Point tenderness to percussion of the spinous processes indicates the possibility of fracture, osteomyelitis, SEA, or malignancy [5,17].

The most important component of the physical examination is the neurologic examination. It is imperative to thoroughly assess motor function, sensation, deep tendon reflexes, gait, and rectal tone. In patients who report urinary incontinence, a postvoid residual should be checked. Acute urinary retention with overflow incontinence can sometimes be the only symptom of neurologic compromise. Any abnormal finding on the neurologic examination suggests the possibility of spinal cord compression. Cord compression is a medical emergency that requires emergent diagnosis and treatment. It is discussed in detail in the following section.

Back pain emergencies

Vascular catastrophes

AD and AAA are two life-threatening vascular disorders that must be considered in the differential diagnosis of the patient who has back pain. Diagnosis of either condition can be challenging because many patients have atypical presentations. The classic textbook presentations of AD and AAA have become the exception rather than the rule. Many patients present with a myriad of complaints attributable to secondary organ involvement. Nonetheless, it is imperative that the internist be able to recognize patients who have these acute aortic emergencies. The mortality for untreated AD is reported to increase 1% to 3% per hour during the first 24 hours of illness [18–20]. For patients who have a rupturing AAA, overall 30-day survival is reported to be as low as 11% despite rapid surgical intervention [16,21].

Aortic dissection

Depending on the study population, the incidence of AD is reported to range from 5 to 30 cases per 1 million population per year [19,22–24]. The diagnosis is missed on initial evaluation in almost 40% of these patients, often due to a combination of factors that include failure to identify significant risk factors, inability to recognize atypical presentations, inattention to physical examination features, and failure to understand the limitations of diagnostic imaging. Common misdiagnoses for AD are acute coronary syndromes, congestive heart failure, pulmonary embolism, musculoskeletal chest pain, musculoskeletal low back strain, cholecystitis, and lumbar radiculopathy [18,25,26].

Failure to assess risk factors is one of the most common reasons cited in litigation for missed AD [18,27]. Male sex, advanced age, and chronic hypertension are well-established risk factors for AD. The incidence of AD is highest among patients between age 50 and 70 years, with a male-to-female ratio in some series as high as 5:1 [18,19,28]. Depending on the population, hypertension is present in nearly 80% of patients who have an AD [19,29]. Other common risk factors include smoking, hyperlipidemia, connective tissue syndromes such as Marfan and Ehlers-Danlos, chromosomal disorders such as Turner's syndrome and Noonan's syndrome, bicuspid aortic valve, coarctation of the aorta, decelerating trauma, inflammatory conditions of the aorta, and aortic instrumentation [19]. Risk factors that are commonly overlooked are pregnancy and the use of cocaine. Cocaine has been shown to predispose patients to AD, particularly of the descending aorta [16,30]. AD in pregnancy occurs most often during the third trimester and the initial stages of labor; 50% of dissections in women less than age 40 years occur during pregnancy [19].

The textbook description of pain in AD is the instantaneous onset of chest pain that is maximal at its onset and is described as knifelike, ripping, or tearing. As stated, this presentation is often the exception rather than the rule. Sharp, knifelike, or tearing pain is only reported in approximately 50% of patients [22]. Location of pain is dependent on the section of aorta that is involved. Dissections of the descending aorta more commonly report back pain than chest pain [26]. Patients who have a descending AD are also more likely to report radiation of pain to the hips and legs, thereby potentially misleading even the seasoned clinician. Aside from the description and location of pain, more than one third of patients present with symptoms attributable to secondary organ involvement [31]. Neurologic symptoms are reported in 18% to 30% of patients who have an AD [19,32,33]. Although signs of cerebral ischemia are more common, symptoms due to spinal cord ischemia are present in up to 10% [19,32]. These patients may present with quadriplegia, paraplegia, or unilateral parasthesias. Thus, any patient who has back pain and neurologic symptoms must still be evaluated for an AD. Additional symptoms of AD include syncope, abdominal pain, gastro-intestinal bleeding, dysphagia, and hoarseness.

Physical examination findings in patients who have suspected AD must be interpreted with caution. Although most of these patients are hypertensive, up to 25% have systolic blood pressures less than 90 mm Hg [18,19,34]. Similarly, significant pulse amplitude differentials in the extremities are found in only ap-proximately 40% of patients [19,35]. Bilateral blood pressure measurements are also of limited value. Although a difference of greater than 20 mm Hg is significant, this degree of discrepancy can also be found in up to 20% of nor-mal individuals [18]. Finally, neurologic symptoms such as parasthesias can be transient [18,22]. Thus, a normal physical examination, including vital signs, can be found in patients who have an acute AD.

When AD is suspected, emergent diagnostic imaging must be obtained. Common imaging modalities include chest radiography, CT, MRI, and transesophageal echocardiography. Chest radiography has limited utility in the diagnosis of AD. Overall sensitivity and specificity is 64% and 86%, respectively [36]. In cases of proximal AD, sensitivity is even lower at 47% [36]. Therefore, AD cannot be ruled out based on a normal chest radiography. At most centers, helical CT has become the emergent imaging modality of choice. Diagnostic accuracy for helical CT in the detection of AD approaches 100% [36]. Although the sensitivity and the specificity for MRI range from 95% to 100%, technical limitations such as long study times, restricted patient access, and restricted monitoring limit its use in the emergent setting [19]. In experienced hands, transesophageal echocardi-ography is an acceptable imaging modality because its sensitivity is reported to be as high as 98% [19,37]. The main drawbacks to transesophageal echo-cardiography are the strong dependence on operator skill and the inability to visualize the aorta below the celiac axis.

Office-based management of the patient who has suspected AD is limited. The most important component is to arrange immediate transfer to the clos-est emergency department. Emergency medical services should be activated and the patient transported according to advanced cardiac life support pro-tocols. While awaiting transfer, intravenous access should be obtained and the patient should be placed on a cardiac monitor. Intravenous antihyper-tensive therapy can be given but should not delay rapid transport. At the present time, standard medical therapy includes the combination of a β-blocker and a vasodilator. Labetolol is recognized as an acceptable al-ternative to combination therapy. Finally, the receiving facility should be notified so as to prepare the appropriate resources.

Abdominal aortic aneurysm

It is estimated that over 1 million Americans have an AAA [38]. It is un-doubtedly a disease of aging because 4% to 8% of individuals over age 65 years are thought to have an AAA [39]. For each decade beyond 65 years, the prevalence of AAA increases by 2% to 4% [40]. Forty percent to 50% of patients who have a rupturing AAA die before reaching medical interven-tion [39]. For the remaining patients who are able to make it to medical treatment, overall mortality exceeds 50% [41]. As with AD, the most impor-tant step in diagnosing AAA is to first consider the diagnosis. Reasons cited for missed AAA are similar to those for AD and include failure to assess risk factors, failure to recognize atypical presentations, and false assurance based on a normal physical examination [18].

Important risk factors for AAA are male sex, advanced age, and hyper-tension. One of the strongest independent risk factors for AAA is smoking [16]. Almost 90% of patients who have an AAA report a history of tobacco use. Additional risk factors are hyperlipidemia, atherosclerotic vascular dis-ease, diabetes, connective tissue disorders, and a family history of AAA. Pa-tients who have a significant family history have a 30% increased risk of developing an AAA [42]. These patients tend to develop aneurysms at an earlier age that are more prone to rupture than those found in patients who do not have a family history of disease [16]. Even though men are 10 times more likely to be affected, AAA must still be considered in a woman who has back pain [43]. For women, rupture occurs three times more fre-quently and at smaller aortic diameters [16].

The textbook triad of hypotension, abdominal pain, and a pulsatile mass occurs in less than 50% of patients who have a rupturing AAA [44]. Patients more commonly present with back pain, left lower-quadrant pain, flank pain, syncope, or lower-extremity parasthesias. As a result, up to 12% of pa-tients are initially misdiagnosed as having diverticulitis [18,45]. Another common misdiagnosis is renal colic due to the fact that 10% of patients have associated urologic symptoms. Although uncommon, AAA can pro-duce neurologic symptoms. Patients may complain of parasthesias of the an-terior thigh or weakness of the hip flexors secondary to aneurysm compression of the femoral or obturator nerves [18].

Physical examination findings that suggest the possibility of an AAA are a palpable pulsatile mass, an abdominal bruit, diminished lower-extremity pulses, and a tender left lower-quadrant mass [18]. The utility of these find-ings in patients who have a rupturing AAA, however, is limited. Overall sen-sitivity is reported to range from 45% to 97% [41]. For those at greatest risk of rupture (aortic diameter >5 cm), 25% of aortas cannot be palpated [18,41]. Sensitivity is further limited in overweight or obese individuals.

Similar to AD, office-based management of a rupturing AAA is limited. Immediate activation of emergency medical services with transport to the closest emergency department is required. Transport and treatment should not be delayed to obtain confirmatory diagnostic imaging. Patients should be placed on a cardiac monitor and intravenous access obtained. In the case of hypotension, isotonic crystalloid fluids should be administered. As with AD, the receiving facility should be notified so that emergent resources can be mobilized.

Malignancy

Approximately 0.7% of patients who have back pain and present to an office-based physician have metastatic cancer [1]. According to the American Cancer Society, over 1.35 million new cases of cancer were diagnosed in 2004, over half of which were malignancies known to metastasize to the spine [46]. Over the same period, 17,000 new cases of primary bone malignancies were diagnosed [47].

Back pain can frequently be the presenting symptom for cancer. Persistent pain, pathologic fracture, and spinal cord compression with permanent neurologic dysfunction can result if the diagnosis is missed.

Cancers that are commonly associated with spinal metastases include breast, prostate, lung, kidney, and thyroid. Breast, prostate, and lung cancer each account for 15% to 20% of cases [48]. Additional malignancies that can metastasize to the spine include non-Hodgkin's lymphoma, multiple myeloma, colorectal carcinoma, and sarcoma [48]. The most common site of malignant spinal lesions is the thoracic spine, accounting for 60% of cases [48]. Lumbosacral involvement is seen in 30% of patients, with cervical lesions accounting for the remaining 10% [49].

Red flags from the history that should raise suspicion for malignancy include age over 50 years, insidious onset of pain, unexplained weight loss, pain that awakens the patient at night, pain that persists despite appropriate therapy, and any previous history of malignancy [8,9,50]. Of these, the strongest risk factor is a prior history of malignancy. Physical examination findings that indicate the possibility of cancer include generalized loss of muscle mass, lymphadenopathy, tenderness to percussion of the spinous processes, and focal neurologic signs [51]. When the diagnosis is suspected, further evaluation is necessary, which most often entails a combination of laboratory and diagnostic imaging studies.

Laboratory studies useful in the diagnosis of malignancy include the erythrocyte sedimentation rate (ESR), complete blood count (CBC), and serum calcium level. The findings of an elevated ESR, hypercalcemia, anemia, and thrombocytopenia indicate the possibility of malignancy. It is reported that the ESR may be the most useful screening test for cancer as an etiology of back pain [50,52,53]. Caution must be used, however, in interpreting an elevated ESR. It is an acute-phase reactant and is elevated in many clinical scenarios such as infection and inflammation. Therefore, an elevated ESR is not specific for the diagnosis of malignancy.

Imaging modalities used in the evaluation for suspected malignancy include plain radiography, CT, radionuclide scanning, and MRI. Given is accessibility and low cost, plain radiography is often chosen as the initial imaging modality. Findings on plain radiography that indicate malignancy are compression fractures, blastic lesions, and lytic lesions. It is unfortunate that plain films are not sensitive or specific for malignancy. In a systematic review, Jarvik and Deyo [46,50] found that a lytic or blastic lesion was only 60% sensitive for cancer. Additional limitations to plain films are the inability to evaluate soft tissue structures and the relatively high dose of radiation to pelvic and gonadal tissues.

The remaining imaging modalities have varying sensitivities and specificities for malignancy. MRI is perhaps the best imaging modality for malignancy, with sensitivity ranging from 83% to 100% [46]. Advantages to MRI include excellent delineation of soft tissue structures with no exposure to ionizing radiation. Although overall inferior to MRI, CT is the study of choice when details regarding cortical structure are required. Available radionuclide scanning techniques include planar radioisotope bone scanning (RBS), single photon emission CT (SPECT), and positron emission tomography. As technology continues to improve, it seems as though SPECT is replacing RBS at most centers. In their review, Jarvik and Deyo [46] reported the sensitivity of SPECT for the detection of cancer to be 87% to 93%. In addition to sensitivity, the specificity of SPECT is improved over that of planar RBS and ranges from 91% to 93% [46].

Management of the patient who has back pain secondary to malignancy hinges on the presence of neurologic symptoms. For those who have evidence of spinal cord compression, emergent treatment is necessary. Treatment of spinal cord compression is discussed in the following section. For those who do not have evidence of compression, treatment comprises a multidisciplinary approach, which most often includes consultation with an oncologist, a radiation oncologist, and an orthopedic surgeon. Hypercalcemia should be aggressively treated with intravenous fluids and bisphosphonates. In a 2003 meta-analysis, Ross and colleagues [54] found that bisphosphonates significantly reduced skeletal morbidity and recommended initiating treatment after the discovery of skeletal metastases. In the absence of neurologic symptoms, steroid administration is controversial. At present, there are no concise recommendations regarding steroids in the absence of neurologic symptoms. Finally, treatment of the patient who has metastatic spinal lesions must include measures for pain relief. If pain is not relieved with traditional analgesic medication, referral to a pain center is indicated.

Spinal cord compression syndromes

Epidural spinal cord compression (ESCC) is defined as radiologic evidence of indentation of the thecal sac [55,56]. Approximately 85% to 90% of cases of ESCC are due to SEM [56]. Less common etiologies include SEA, spinal epidural hematoma, and central disc herniation. Disc herniation resulting in compression below the termination of the spinal cord is termed the cauda equina syndrome. Cauda equina syndrome is grouped with other causes of ESCC because the pathophysiology is identical to compression at higher levels. The incidence of ESCC varies according to etiology. Cauda equina syndrome complicates approximately 2% of cases of lumbar disc herniation [57]. ESCC due to SEM is reported to occur in 5% of patients who have cancer [56,58]; 20% of cases of ESCC are the initial manifestation of malignancy [59]. Spinal epidural hematoma is a rare disorder with no reliable published data on the incidence of disease. SEA is discussed in detail in the subsequent section.

Risk factors for ESCC are numerous. Because most cases are caused by SEM, primary risk factors are the same as those previously discussed for malignancy. Patients who abuse intravenous drugs, have recently had a bacterial infection, or have undergone a procedure known to cause bacteremia are at risk of ESCC secondary to SEA. ESCC due to spinal epidural hematoma almost exclusively occurs in patients receiving anticoagulation therapy. Thus, a thorough review of medications is necessary.

Clinical features of ESCC consist primarily of back pain and neurologic impairment. Pain is reported in 83% to 95% of patients and usually precedes neurologic symptoms by an average of 7 weeks [49,58,60,61]. The description and characteristics of back pain vary and depend on the location of the lesion. Some patients report severe localized thoracic pain, whereas others may describe unilateral lumbar pain with radiation to the ipsilateral lower extremity. It is unfortunate that many cases of ESCC are not diagnosed until the onset of neurologic symptoms. The average delay in diagnosis from the onset of back pain is 2 to 3 months [61,62]. Predominant neurologic symptoms of ESCC are motor weakness, parasthesias, bowel and bladder dysfunction, and gait abnormalities. Motor weakness is the most common symptom, affecting 60% to 85% of patients at the time of diagnosis [61,62]. Although virtually any pattern of muscle weakness can be seen, ESCC typically causes symmetric lower-extremity findings [61]. For lesions involving the spinal cord, hyper-reflexia is seen below the level of compression. In the case of cauda equina syndrome, however, hyporeflexia is the typical finding. Sensory abnormalities occur less commonly and include bilateral ascending parasthesias, saddle anesthesia, and unilateral parasthesias in a radicular pattern. Any patient who reports saddle anesthesia should be considered to have cauda equina syndrome until proved otherwise. Bowel or bladder dysfunction is frequently a late finding of cord compression. Nonetheless, acute urinary retention with overflow incontinence may be the initial (and only) finding of ESCC. Any report of urinary retention mandates that a postvoid residual be checked.

When ESCC is considered, emergent diagnostic imaging must be obtained. As stated, ESCC requires radiographic confirmation of indentation of the thecal sac. Available imaging modalities include plain radiography, radionuclide bone scan, CT, myelography, and MRI. Plain films are inadequate in the diagnosis of ESCC because 10% to 17% of patients who have ESCC have normal plain films [49,58,61]. Similarly, radionuclide bone scans and CT are of limited value in diagnosing ESCC. Although both modalities can provide information regarding spinal metastases, neither can clearly image the spinal cord or epidural space. The two definitive imaging modalities for ESCC are myelography and MRI. Myelography is an invasive technique in which contrast is injected directly into the thecal sac. CT can be combined with myelography to provide added anatomic detail. Myelography can be performed relatively quickly and has the added benefit of cerebrospinal fluid analysis. Despite these advantages, myelography is being replaced by MRI at many institutions. In addition to diagnosing ESCC, MRI can provide information regarding masses that are not compressing the spine [63,64]. For patients who have contraindications to MRI, myelography remains the imaging modality of choice.

ESCC is a medical emergency that requires immediate treatment. Although treatment algorithms are based on specific etiologies, nearly all implement a multidisciplinary approach. Most often, this approach involves emergent orthopedic or neurosurgical consultation. For patients who have cauda equina syndrome, early lumbar laminectomy with discectomy has been shown to improve outcome [57,65]. Ahn and colleagues [66] reported significant improvement in motor, sensory, urinary, and rectal symptoms when decompression was performed within 48 hours. Patients who have SEA and signs of compression require surgical drainage. In addition, patients should be started on broad-spectrum antibiotics while awaiting intervention. Depending on the size and location of the abscess, drainage can sometimes be accomplished by an interventional radiologist. Management of the patient who has ESCC secondary to SEM requires consultation with a radiation oncologist in addition to the surgical subspecialties. Frequently, radiotherapy alone results in improvement in symptoms. Patients who have malignant spinal cord compression should be given systemic steroids. High-dose steroids have been reported to improve rates of postradiation ambulation [67]. Steroid administration for nonmalignant spinal cord compression is controversial and remains a current topic of debate.

Infectious etiologies

Overall, infectious causes of back pain are uncommon. Nevertheless, these conditions must be considered because any delay in diagnosis or treatment may result in potentially disastrous complications. Vertebral osteomyelitis and SEA are two infectious etiologies of back pain that, when undiagnosed, can result in permanent neurologic dysfunction or death. Although discussed separately, it is important to understand that these entities are likely part of a continuum of infection.

Vertebral osteomyelitis

Vertebral osteomyelitis is defined as the inflammation of a vertebral body due to a pyogenic organism. Frequently, the infection spreads to the

adjacent disc space, resulting in a spondylodiscitis. Despite the relative paucity of published information, many authorities believe that the incidence of
vertebral osteomyelitis is increasing [68]. Most cite the aging population, the
increasing use of injection drugs, and the increasing rates of bacteremia secondary to indwelling devices as explanations for the increased incidence [68].
Gram-positive cocci, namely *Staphylococcus aureus*, account for most of the
pyogenic organisms that cause vertebral osteomyelitis. Depending on the
patient population, other organisms include gram-negative bacilli such as
Pseudomonas aeruginosa, various *Candida* species, *Salmonella*, and *Myco-
bacterium tuberculosis* [69,70]. More commonly, these organisms cause osteomyelitis as a result of hematogenous spread from a distant focus. Other,
less common sources of infection are contiguous spread from an adjacent
infection and direct inoculation from a medical procedure [68].

Most patients who have vertebral osteomyelitis present with back pain
[71]. As discussed, back pain due to osteomyelitis typically presents in an in-
dolent fashion over a period of weeks to months. The location of pain can
be anywhere along the spine, although the thoracic and lumbar areas are
more commonly involved [71,72]. Physical examination usually reveals tenderness to percussion of the spinous process of the involved vertebral body.
Although a thorough neurologic examination is necessary, significant deficits are found in less than 20% of patients who have vertebral osteomyelitis
[71,73]. Patient temperature must be interpreted with caution. It is well
known that patients who have vertebral osteomyelitis are frequently afebrile
[68,71,74]. Thus, the lack of fever is insufficient evidence to rule out the
diagnosis.

Laboratory studies frequently obtained in the patient who has suspected
osteomyelitis include blood cultures, CBC, ESR, and C-reactive protein. Because the most frequent mode of infection is hematogenous spread, blood
cultures should be obtained in every patient. Depending on the study, cultures are positive in up to 70% of patients and can help guide antibiotic
therapy [68,69,75]. Similarly, wound cultures should be obtained on any purulent soft tissue infection because this may be the nidus of infection. The
CBC is less helpful. Leukocytosis is present in less than half of patients
who have osteomyelitis [71–73,76]. A normal white blood cell count should
never be used as sole criteria to exclude osteomyelitis. ESR and C-reactive
protein are reportedly more sensitive for the detection of osteomyelitis.
Both are acute-phase reactants and, in the case of osteomyelitis, often markedly elevated. Some investigators have used ESR and C-reactive protein to
follow response to therapy, but this methodology remains a topic of debate
in the medical literature.

Imaging modalities used for the diagnosis of osteomyelitis include plain
radiography, radionuclide bone scan, CT, and MRI. Often, the initial imaging modality is plain radiography. Abnormalities that are consistent with
osteomyelitis include erosion of the vertebral endplate, lytic bony abnormalities, disc space narrowing, and possibly prevertebral soft tissue swelling

[71,77]. Unfortunately, these abnormalities can take several weeks to become evident, thereby limiting the utility of plain films. Radionuclide bone scanning is reported to have good sensitivity for detecting infection [68,71,78]. Sensitivity and specificity are highest when using gallium scintigraphy. An advantage to bone scanning is the ability to detect additional areas of infection; however, disadvantages are numerous and include false-positive and false-negative results and the inability to provide anatomic detail. MRI is the diagnostic modality of choice in suspected osteomyelitis or spondylodiscitis [71,77,78]. Even early in the disease process, MRI demonstrates signs of edema and inflammation. Additional advantages include the ability to determine the extent of disease and spinal cord involvement. Helical CT can be used in cases in which MRI is unavailable. Limitations to CT are a relatively low specificity and a high false-negative rate of detecting complications such as epidural abscess.

Most patients can be successfully treated with antibiotic therapy alone. In the absence of neurologic symptoms, most investigators recommend obtaining tissue samples before the initiation of antimicrobial therapy. This process can often be accomplished through CT-guided needle biopsy. Antibiotics should be broad spectrum and given intravenously until a clinical response is seen. Duration of antibiotics is dependent on clinical response but usually ranges from 6 to 12 weeks. Indications for operative intervention include the presence of a fluid collection, impending cord compression, and progression of disease despite adequate antimicrobial coverage. Adjunctive therapy includes spinal immobilization and long-acting analgesics.

Spinal epidural abscess

SEA comprises 0.2 to 2 cases per 10,000 hospital admissions [79]. As stated, SEA is part of a continuum of infection that often develops as a result of untreated spondylodiscitis. Patients at any age can be affected. There have been case reports of SEA in patients as young as 10 days and as old as 87 years [79]. SEA more commonly affects the thoracic and lumbar spine but can occur at any spinal level [71]. Furthermore, extension of the abscess is common. The average extent of an abscess spans 3 to 5 spinal cord segments [80]. Gram-positive organisms, namely *Staphylococcus aureus*, account for most of the organisms isolated in SEA. Although the most common portal of entry is from skin and soft tissue infections, up to one third are due to hematogenous spread. Injection drug use is the most common risk factor for hematogenous seeding of the spine [81].

The classic clinical triad of SEA is fever, back pain, and neurologic deficits. Unfortunately, this triad is present in less than 20% of patients [82]. Clearly, back pain is the most common complaint of an SEA. The pain tends to be severe and is usually localized to the midline. Tenderness to percussion of the spinous process is a common physical examination finding. Although it is written that patients are usually febrile and appear ill, many are normothermic or have only modest degrees of temperature elevation [71]. The absence of fever should never dissuade the physician from considering the diagnosis. Neurologic symptoms are present in many patients and include motor weakness, parasthesias, and bowel or bladder dysfunction. Up to 35% of patients have bowel or bladder incontinence at the time of presentation [71]. The presence of neurologic findings is foreboding. Patients can rapidly progress to complete paralysis, which when present, is usually irreversible.

Laboratory studies commonly ordered in the evaluation of SEA include blood cultures, CBC, and ESR. All patients should have blood cultures drawn because there is excellent correlation with organisms obtained from the abscess [71]. Although not helpful acutely, culture results help guide antibiotic therapy during the course of hospitalization. The utility of the CBC is limited because many patients who have an SEA do not have a leukocytosis [71,82]. Thus, a normal white blood cell count is insufficient to rule out the diagnosis. An elevated ESR is common in cases of SEA, but ESR is also elevated in a number of other disease states and, therefore, is not specific for SEA. In some cases, the ESR can be used to guide therapy because it has been shown to correlate with disease resolution [71].

MRI is the imaging modality of choice when evaluating a patient for an SEA. MRI has been shown to be accurate in identifying the abscess, defining the extent of disease, and determining the presence of thecal sac compression [71]. When MRI is not available or is contraindicated, CT myelography is an acceptable alternative; however, it is an invasive procedure with increased risks. Plain films are inadequate in the diagnosis of SEA. Although signs such as endplate erosion can suggest the diagnosis, many patients who have an SEA have nonspecific or even normal findings [71].

The mainstay of therapy for the patient who has an SEA is surgical decompression and drainage. Ideally, this should be accomplished within 24 hours of presentation. Any significant delay in therapy can result in permanent paraplegia or incontinence. All patients require hospitalization for initiation of treatment. As with most back pain emergencies, treatment of an SEA requires a multidisciplinary approach. Immediate consultation with a neurosurgeon is warranted. Consultation with an orthopedic surgeon, infectious disease specialist, and interventional radiologist is also recommended. In cases in which the SEA is small, aspiration and drainage can sometimes be accomplished with CT-guided techniques alone. Broad-spectrum antibiotic therapy covering gram-positive and gram-negative bacilli should be initiated. Duration of antibiotic therapy depends on the clinical situation but usually lasts from 4 to 6 weeks.

Summary

Most adults in the United States will experience an episode of back pain at some point during their lifetime. Most will present to their primary care physician for evaluation and treatment. Many patients have non–life-threatening etiologies and recover within 4 to 6 weeks. A small percentage, however, have back pain due to a potentially life-threatening emergency. AD, rupturing AAA, SEM, cauda equina syndrome, vertebral osteomyelitis, and SEA are just some of the medical emergencies that can present with back pain. Clinical suspicion for these diagnoses begins with a thorough history and physical examination. It is imperative that the office-based physician search for and accurately identify any red flag within the history or physical examination. Appropriate laboratory studies and diagnostic imaging are obtained based on the suspected etiology.

References

[1] Mazanec D. Back pain: medical evaluation and therapy. Cleve Clin J Med 1995;62:163–8.
[2] Kelsey JL, White AA III. Epidemiology and impact of low-back pain. Spine 1980;5:133–42.
[3] Koes BW, Assendelft WJ, van der Heijden GJ, et al. Spinal manipulation for low back pain. An updated systematic review of randomized clinical trials. Spine 1996;21:2860–73.
[4] Humphreys SC, Eck JC, Hodges SD. Radiologic decision-making: neuroimaging in low back pain. Am Fam Physician 2002;65(11):2299–306.
[5] Della-Gustina DA. Orthopedic emergencies: emergency department evaluation and treatment of back pain. Emerg Med Clin North Am 1999;17(4):877–93.
[6] Praemer A, Furner S, Rice D. Musculoskeletal conditions in the United States. In: Proceedings of the American Academy of Orthopedic Surgeons. Rosemont (IL): AAOS; 1992. p. 23–33.
[7] Hart LG, Deyo RA, Cherkin DC. Physician office visits for low back pain: frequency, clinical evaluation, and treatment patterns from a US national survey. Spine 1995;20:11–9.
[8] Deyo RA, Weinstein JN. Low back pain. N Engl J Med 2001;344:363–70.
[9] Bigos S, Bowyer O, Braen G, et al. Acute low back problems in adults. Clinical practice guideline, quick reference number 14. Rockville (MD): US Department of Health and Human Services, Public Health Service, Agency for Health Care Policy and Research; 1994. Publication #AHCPR 95–0643.
[10] Hanley E. Distinguishing the specific from the non-specific low back pain. Bull Hosp Joint Dis 1996;55:195–6.
[11] Devereaux MW. Low back pain. Prim Care Clin Office Pract 2004;31(1):33–51.
[12] Levin KH, Covington EC, Devereaux MW, et al. Neck and low back pain. Continuum (N Y) 2001;7:1–205.
[13] Malcolm J. Acute back pain. Clin Med 2001;1(3):188–9.
[14] Lehrich JR, Katz JN, Sheon RP. Approach to the diagnosis and evaluation of low back pain in adults. Available at: http://www.uptodate.com. Accessed 2004.
[15] Schmidt R, Markovchick V. Nontraumatic spinal cord compression. J Emerg Med 1992;10: 189–99.
[16] Isselbacher EM. Thoracic and abdominal aortic aneurysms. Circulation 2005;111(6): 816–28.
[17] Deyo R, Rainville J, Kent D. What can the history and physical examination tell us about low back pain. JAMA 1992;286:760–5.
[18] Rogers RL, McCormack R. Aortic disasters. Emerg Med Clin North Am 2004;22(4): 887–908.
[19] Khan IA, Nair CK. Clinical, diagnostic, and management perspectives of aortic dissection. Chest 2002;122(1):311–28.

[20] Pitt MP, Bonser RS. The natural history of thoracic aortic aneurysm disease: an overview. J Card Surg 1997;12:270–8.

[21] Brown PM, Pattenden R, Vernooy C, et al. Selective management of abdominal aortic aneurysms in a prospective measurement program. J Vasc Surg 1996;23:213–20.

[22] Hagan PG, Nienaber CA, Isselbacher EM, et al. The International Registry of Acute Aortic Dissection (IRAD): new insights into an old disease. JAMA 2000;283:897–903.

[23] Eisenberg MJ, Rice SA, Paraschos A, et al. The clinical spectrum of patients with aneurysms of the ascending aorta. Am Heart J 1993;125:1380–5.

[24] Bickerstaff LK, Pairolero PC, Hoiler LH, et al. Thoracic aortic aneurysms: a population based study. Surgery 1982;92:1103–8.

[25] Spittel PC, Spittel JA, Joyce JW, et al. Clinical features and differential diagnosis of aortic dissection: experience with 236 cases. Mayo Clin Proc 1993;68:642–51.

[26] Nienaber CA, Eagle KA. Aortic dissection: new frontiers in diagnosis and management. Part I: from etiology to diagnostic strategies. Circulation 2003;108(5):628–35.

[27] Sullivan D. Thoracic aortic dissection: medical error and risk reduction. In: High-risk acute care: the failure to diagnose. The Sullivan Group 1997. Available at: http://www.thesullivangroup.com.

[28] Auer J, Berent R, Eber B. Aortic dissection: incidence, natural history and impact of surgery. J Clin Basic Cardiol 2000;3:151–4.

[29] Hennessy TG, Smith D, McCann HA, et al. Thoracic aortic dissection or aneurysm: clinical presentation, diagnostic imaging and initial management in a tertiary referral center. Ir J Med Sci 1996;165:259–62.

[30] Hsue PY, Salinas CL, Bolger AF, et al. Acute aortic dissection related to crack cocaine. Circulation 2002;105:592–5.

[31] Khan IA. Clinical manifestations of aortic dissection. J Clin Basic Cardiol 2001;4:265–7.

[32] Alverez Sabin J, Vazquez J, Sala A, et al. Neurologic manifestations of dissecting aneurysm of the aorta. Med Clin (Barc) 1989;92:447–9.

[33] Prendes JL. Neurovascular syndromes in aortic dissection. Am Fam Physician 1981;23: 175–9.

[34] Garcia-Jiminez A, Paraza-Torres A, Martinez-Lopez G, et al. Cardiac tamponade by aortic dissection in a hospital without cardiothoracic surgery. Chest 1993;104:290–1.

[35] von Kodolitsch Y, Schwartz AG, Nienaber CA. Clinical prediction of acute aortic dissection. Arch Intern Med 2000;160:2977–82.

[36] Higgins CB. Modern imaging of the acute aortic syndrome. Am J Med 2004;116:134.

[37] Vignon P, Gueret, Vedrinne JM, et al. Role of transesophageal echocardiography in the diagnosis and management of traumatic aortic disruption. Circulation 1995;92: 2959–68.

[38] Hallet JW. Management of abdominal aortic aneurysms. Mayo Clin Proc 2000;74:395–9.

[39] Beebe HG, Kritpracha B. Screening and preoperative imaging of candidates for conventional repair of abdominal aortic aneurysm. Semin Vasc Surg 1999;12:300–5.

[40] Powell JT, Greenhalgh RM. Small abdominal aortic aneurysms. N Engl J Med 2003;348: 1895–901.

[41] Carpenter CR. Abdominal palpation for the diagnosis of abdominal aortic aneurysm. Ann Emerg Med 2005;45:556–7.

[42] Frydam G, Walker PJ, Summers K, et al. The value of screening in siblings of patients with abdominal aortic aneurysm. Eur J Vasc Endovasc Surg 2003;26:396–400.

[43] Lederle FA, Johnson GR, Wilson SE. Aneurysm detection and management. Veterans Affairs Cooperative Study: abdominal aortic aneurysm in women. J Vasc Surg 2001;34: 122–6.

[44] Steele MA, Dalsing MC. Emergency evaluation of abdominal aortic aneurysm. Indiana Med 1987;80:862–4.

[45] Marston WA, Ahlquist R, Johnson G, et al. Misdiagnosis of ruptured abdominal aortic aneurysms. J Vasc Surg 1992;16:17–22.

[46] Jarvik JG, Deyo RA. Diagnostic evaluation of low back pain with emphasis on imaging. Ann Intern Med 2002;137:586–97.

[47] American Cancer Society. Cancer facts and figures 2004. Available at: http://www.cancer. org. Accessed December 1, 2005.

[48] Schiff D. Spinal cord compression. Neurol Clin N Am 2003;21:67–86.

[49] Posner JB. Neurologic complications of cancer. Philadelphia: FA Davis; 1995.

[50] Deyo RA, Diehl AK. Cancer as a cause of back pain: frequency, clinical presentation, and diagnostic strategies. J Gen Intern Med 1988;3:230–8.

[51] Atlas SJ, Nardin RA. Evaluation and treatment of low back pain: an evidence-based approach to clinical care. Muscle Nerve 2003;27:265–84.

[52] Deyo RA. Early diagnostic evaluation of low back pain. J Gen Intern Med 1986;1: 328–38.

[53] van den Hoogen HM, Koes BW, van Eijk JT, et al. On the accuracy of history, physical examination, and erythrocyte sedimentation rate in diagnosing low back pain in general practice. A criteria based review of the literature. Spine 1995;20:318–27.

[54] Ross JR, Saunders Y, Edmonds PM, et al. Systematic review of role of bisphosphonates on skeletal morbidity in metastatic cancer. BMJ 2003;327:469.

[55] Loblaw DA, Perry J, Chambers A, et al. Systematic review of the diagnosis and management of malignant extradural spinal cord compression: the Cancer Care Ontario Practice Guidelines Initiative's Neuro-Oncology Disease Site Group. J Clin Oncol 2005;23:2028–37.

[56] Schiff D, O'Neill BP, Wang CH, et al. Neuroimaging and treatment implications of patients with multiple epidural spinal metastases. Cancer 1998;83:1593–601.

[57] Kostuik JP, Harrington I, Alexander D, et al. Cauda equina syndrome and lumbar disc herniation. J Bone Joint Surg Am 1986;68:386–91.

[58] Bach F, Larsen BH, Rohde K, et al. Metastatic spinal cord compression. Occurrence, symptoms, clinical presentations and prognosis in 398 patients with spinal cord compression. Acta Neurochir (Wien) 1990;107:37–43.

[59] Schiff D, O'Neill BP, Suman VJ. Spinal epidural metastasis as the initial manifestation of malignancy: clinical features and diagnostic approach. Neurology 1997;49:52–6.

[60] Helweg-Larsen S, Sorenson PS. Symptoms and signs in metastatic spinal cord compression: a study of progression from first symptom until diagnosis in 153 patients. Eur J Cancer 1994; 30A:396–8.

[61] Schiff D. Clinical features and diagnosis of epidural spinal cord compression, including cauda equina syndrome. Available at: www.uptodate.com. Accessed October 2003.

[62] Husband DJ. Malignant spinal cord compression: prospective study of delays in referral and treatment. BMJ 1998;317:18–21.

[63] Carmody RF, Yang PJ, Seeley GW, et al. Spinal cord compression due to metastatic disease: diagnosis with MR imaging versus myelography. Radiology 1989;173:225–9.

[64] Li KC, Poon PY. Sensitivity and specificity of MRI in detecting malignant spinal cord compression and in distinguishing malignant from benign compression fractures of vertebrae. Magn Reson Imaging 1988;6:547–56.

[65] Bartels RH, de Vries J. Hemi-cauda equina syndrome from herniated lumbar disc: a neurosurgical emergency? Can J Neurol Sci 1996;23:296–9.

[66] Ahn UM, Ahn NU, Buchowski JM, et al. Cauda equina syndrome secondary to lumbar disc herniation: a meta-analysis of surgical outcomes. Spine 2000;25:1515–22.

[67] Sorenson S, Helweg-Larsen S, Mouridsen H, et al. Effect of high-dose dexamethasone in carcinomatous metastatic spinal cord compression treated with radiotherapy: a randomized trial. Spine 1994;30A:22–7.

[68] Sexton DJ, McDonald M. Vertebral osteomyelitis. Available at: www.uptodate.com. Accessed January 2005.

[69] Nolla JM, Ariza J, Gomez-Vaquero C, et al. Spontaneous pyogenic vertebral osteomyelitis in nondrug users. Semin Arthritis Rheum 2002;31:271–8.

[70] Lew DP, Waldvogel FA. Osteomyelitis. Lancet 2004;364:369–85.

[71] Calder KK, Severyn FA. Surgical emergencies in the intravenous drug user. Emerg Med Clin North Am 2003;21:1089–116.
[72] Hadjipavlou AG, Mader JT, Necessary JT, et al. Hematogenous pyogenic infections and their surgical management. Spine 2000;25:1668–79.
[73] Sapico FL, Montgomerie JZ. Vertebral osteomyelitis in intravenous drug abusers: report of three cases and review of the literature. Rev Infect Dis 1980;2(2):196–206.
[74] Torda AJ, Gottlieb T, Bradbury R. Pyogenic vertebral osteomyelitis: analysis of 20 cases and review. Clin Infect Dis 1995;20:320–8.
[75] Patzakis MJ, Rao S, Wilkins J, et al. Analysis of 61 cases of vertebral osteomyelitis. Clin Orthop 1991;264:178–83.
[76] Broner FA, Garland DE, Zigler JE. Spinal infections in the immunocompromised host. Orthop Clin North Am 1996;27(1):37–46.
[77] Rothman SL. The diagnosis of infections of the spine by modern imaging techniques. Orthop Clin 1996;27(1):15–31.
[78] Modic MT, Feiglin DH, Piraino DW, et al. Vertebral osteomyelitis: assessment using MR. Radiology 1985;157:157–66.
[79] Reihsaus E, Waldbaur H, Seeling W. Spinal epidural abscess: a meta-analysis of 915 patients. Neurosurg Rev 2000;23(4):175–204.
[80] Darouiche RO, Hamill RJ, Greenberg SB, et al. Bacterial spinal epidural abscess: review of 43 cases and literature survey. Medicine (Baltimore) 1992;17:369–85.
[81] Durack DT, Sexton DJ. Epidural abscess. Available at: www.uptodate.com. Accessed January 2005.
[82] Davis DP, Wold RM, Patel RJ, et al. The clinical presentation and impact of diagnostic delays on emergency department patients with spinal epidural abscess. J Emerg Med 2004;26:285–91.

ELSEVIER
SAUNDERS

THE MEDICAL
CLINICS
OF NORTH AMERICA

Med Clin N Am 90 (2006) 525–532

Index

Note: Page numbers of article titles are in **boldface** type.

0025-7125/06/$ - see front matter © 2006 Elsevier Inc. All rights reserved.
doi:10.1016/S0025-7125(06)00025-3 *medical.theclinics.com*

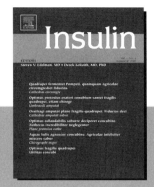

Changing Your Address?

Make sure your subscription changes too! When you notify us of your new address, you can help make our job easier by including an exact copy of your Clinics label number with your old address (see illustration below.) This number identifies you to our computer system and will speed the processing of your address change. Please be sure this label number accompanies your old address and your corrected address—you can send an old Clinics label with your number on it or just copy it exactly and send it to the address listed below.

We appreciate your help in our attempt to give you continuous coverage. Thank you.

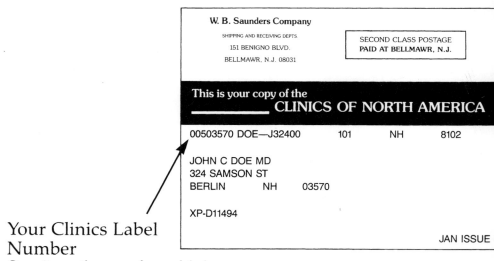

W. B. Saunders Company

SHIPPING AND RECEIVING DEPTS.
151 BENIGNO BLVD.
BELLMAWR, N.J. 08031

SECOND CLASS POSTAGE
PAID AT BELLMAWR, N.J.

This is your copy of the
CLINICS OF NORTH AMERICA

00503570 DOE—J32400   101   NH   8102

JOHN C DOE MD
324 SAMSON ST
BERLIN   NH   03570

XP-D11494

JAN ISSUE

Your Clinics Label Number

Copy it exactly or send your label along with your address to:
W.B. Saunders Company, Customer Service
Orlando, FL 32887-4800
Call Toll Free 1-800-654-2452

Please allow four to six weeks for delivery of new subscriptions and for processing address changes.